CONTENTS

HOLISTIC WEIGHT LOSS

An 8-Week Program To Losing Weight The Healthy
Way Through The Mind and Food

DISCLAIMER

By reading this disclaimer, you are accepting the terms of the disclaimer in full. If you disagree with this disclaimer, please do not read the book. The content in this book is provided for informational and educational purposes only.

This book is not intended to be a substitute for the original work of this diet plan. At most, this All product names, diet plans, or names used in this book are for identification purposes only and are property of their respective owners. Use of these names does not imply endorsement. All other trademarks cited herein are property of their respective owners.

None of the information in this book should be accepted as independent medical or other professional advice.

The information in the books has been compiled from various sources that are deemed reliable. It has been analyzed and summarized to the best of the Author's ability, knowledge, and belief.

However, the Author cannot guarantee the accuracy and thus should not be held liable for any errors.

You acknowledge and agree that the Author of this book will not be held liable for any damages, costs, expenses, resulting from the application of the information in this book, whether directly or indirectly. You acknowledge and agree that you assume all risk and responsibility for any action you undertake in response to the information in this book.

You acknowledge and agree that by continuing to read this book, you will (where applicable, appropriate, or necessary) consult a qualified medical professional on this information. The information in this book is not intended to be any sort of medical advice and should not be used in lieu of any medical advice by a licensed and qualified medical professional.

Always seek the advice of your physician or another qualified health provider with any issues or questions you might have regarding any sort of medical condition. Do not ever disregard any qualified professional medical advice or delay seeking that advice because of anything you have read in this book.

WEEK 1:

THIS IS WHY YOU'RE NOT LOSING WEIGHT—

When it comes to weight loss, many of us tend to be guilty of many different so-called "sins" that we commit in an attempt to shed off the pounds as quickly as possible. However, this urgent mindset actually causes more harm than good. Think back to all the fad diets you've tried before; all those detox teas, various shakes and drinks, as well as magic pills that promised plenty but delivered little to none. In many cases, you ended up gaining all the weight you've lost.

The big question is WHY? Why do you keep failing and why do you keep gaining back the lost weight?

The answer is simple: It's because of your approach towards weight loss. In wanting to quickly lose weight in time for a vacation or a family holiday, you forego considering the bigger picture. You're only thinking about the numbers without giving much thought to your health on a more holistic level. Fact is, the most effective weight loss often comes as a natural result of lifestyle changes and bettering your overall relationship with food.

This is something I learned through experience.

I'VE BEEN IN YOUR SHOES BEFORE.

As a teen, I always had trouble maintaining my ideal weight —there were many factors to blame, but I also lacked proper discipline when it comes to food. Whenever I'd get stressed out, I would turn to eating as a means of relaxing. I would reward myself with food whenever I did great at school, without realizing how detrimental it was towards my health and my performance in classes. I would often feel foggy and lethargic. During afternoon classes, I would easily lose focus and could barely get through the rest of the day if it weren't for caffeine.

I didn't realize that I felt that way because I was eating bad food—the kind that tasted good but did not nourish my body sufficiently. It left me lacking in energy, despite feeling full, and sleepy throughout the day. Instead, I blamed it on my workload or on the fact that I wasn't getting enough sleep. For a time, I even believed that I was anemic! But I never bothered to get myself properly diagnosed, believing that I'd eventually figure it out and things would get better.

However, this continued until after I had graduated school. It began to affect my work performance, causing me to feel restless throughout the day—often craving specific dishes that I would indulge in as soon as I clocked out. Sounds unhealthy, right? Well, that's the kind of relationship I had with food. It made me feel good and so I often wanted it; doesn't matter if the "high" is short-lived. This went on until my mid-twenties, wherein I hit my heaviest weight.

Without realizing it, I was causing more and more damage to my health. The wake-up call was painful, but necessary. I began experiencing joint pains and inflammation in my legs, specifically in my ankles. Until one day, I couldn't even finish walking my pet dogs—that was when it hit me: I was only 25, but my body felt years older. Other people my age were leading active lives; they were going on adventures and seemed to be at the peak of their health. Meanwhile, here I was, unable to walk the half-block home because of the pain in my legs.

You might be familiar with this; how we sometimes end up on auto-pilot day in and day out. Not living mindfully as we should and falling into routines, and bad habits without fully realizing its consequences. We eat take-out everyday because it's convenient. After a long day of working, who wants to bother with cooking? But it's these small things that matter the most when it comes to maintaining holistic health.

This, among other things, will be tackled throughout this course. As we go through each module, you will be provided with actionable steps and assignments to help you put everything you learn into practice. It is one thing to read something from a book and a whole other challenge trying to actually live it. Before we jump into the next phase, however, I request that forget about what you think you know about losing weight. You must let go of your biases and keep an open mind throughout this journey.

THE RESET: RELEARNING, RESTARTING.

If you are among the many others who have unsuccessfully tried to lose weight before, then you're well aware of just how much information is out there about the subject. There's so much, in fact, that you can easily find yourself overwhelmed—unsure of where or how to start. In this course, I did the legwork on your behalf; going through various health resources, from books to websites, and testing out what works and what doesn't. Needless to say, what you're getting here is a compilation of all the useful content I have discovered. We're talking concise information, to make sure you get the proper guidance you need when it comes to your weight loss journey.

See, this is one of the most common issues that many dieters face: THE LACK OF DIRECTION.

Think of weight loss as a ladder. Each step is important in order for you to reach your goal and should you skip one, you risk falling back to the very beginning. This is why it's also imperative that you know exactly which steps to take. By having a clear idea of what's ahead, you will no longer feel lost and be tempted to give up on your weight loss journey.

So now, we begin with a blank slate. This is where a MENTALITY SHIFT needs to happen. Throughout your weight loss journey, you must have gathered countless information about nutrition and various aspects to losing weight. Some are solid facts, whilst most are likely to be non-scientific myths that you were told in order for companies to sell more of their products. Perhaps you've also come to believe that the reason you're not losing weight is because you aren't doing enough. You're either:

Not exercising enough

Not following the food restrictions properly

Not counting your calories strictly

Not eating the right kind of food

And so on. You might have been even led to believe that you have bad genetics—therefore, you can't really do much else about your weight. I empathize with you when it comes to feeling hopeless at times. I have been there myself; moments in the past where I simply gave up because nothing seems to be working. Not the hours I spent in the gym or the meals I skipped in order to lose a few pounds. After all, if the popular diets aren't working for me, then there must be something wrong with my body—right? Wrong. Truth was, I simply didn't have the right mindset to make them work for me. I was accepting all the information I read as fact, without really digging further into it.

This greatly compromised my progress and it might be happening to you, too.

TWO MAJOR ISSUES ENCOUNTERED BY DIETERS.

First: It might surprise you to learn that MANY of the current information we're being fed when it comes to weight loss is severely outdated. This is why a lot of people still believe common misconceptions about fats being unhealthy and that simply eating them will make you fat. Science says there's very little truth to this and later on, you'll learn that fats can be an important part of your everyday diet—even whilst you're dieting.

Are you ready for a plot twist? WHEAT is one of the biggest reasons why people gain weight—not FAT, which so many people are afraid of.

Second: Another common issue is that a lot of the available diet programs and plans don't always address the root cause of a person's obesity as well as their chronic health issues. Sure, losing weight is great, but that's just one part of the problem. This is why you need a holistic solution; something that will tackle the issue from its root and bring about overall healing. Ask yourself this question: With the amount of weight loss information available for free, why are the statistics for obesity still alarmingly high? The numbers don't lie. 68% of Americans are either obese or overweight with numbers increasing across the globe as well.

Let's break down the global statistics:

30% of the world's population is obese—that's equal to 2 million people who are suffering from its ill effects.

The obesity rates in about 70 different countries have doubled since the 1980's and it isn't just adults who are affected by it. Childhood obesity rates have also increased exponentially, much faster than the adult obesity rate.

There are over 340 million children, as well as adolescents, who are overweight or obese.

In a report made by TIME magazine, several factors have been pointed out as major contributors to this epidemic. This includes larger food portions, easy access to fast food, and the habitual consumption of processed food.

Obesity is, in fact, linked to more deaths globally when compared to a person being underweight. Today, there are more obese people than those who are underweight— a phenomena that occurs in every region except certain parts of Asia and sub-Saharan Africa.

So, does this mean that this percentage of the world population isn't trying hard enough? Or are their efforts simply being rendered futile because the methods they are using doesn't get to the core of the issue?

FACT: Obesity is also a mental problem.

It can be a hard pill to swallow for some, especially the ones who still believe that they have full control over their weights and their eating problem. I was one of those people, too, until I realized that I had zero control over what I was doing and that food has become an addiction—one that I was constantly feeding. But, see, it's this lack of awareness that makes it difficult to tackle. Few people take the time to understand and assess their relationship with food and why they eat so much unhealthy stuff. Instead, they soothe their guilty conscience with a new diet program or book; something they will read and feel motivated by, only to fall back into old habits without having put the knowledge they gained into action.

In this case, however, it isn't always your fault. These books tend to bombard people with information without really presenting a clear cut process of what needs to be done. Instead, most diet books go on and on about the science of weight loss—basically, the things that people don't really care about. This isn't to say that there are no programs that would provide you with a concise guide towards achieving your ideal weight; there are ones available online but they will cost you thousands of dollars.

THE PROBLEM WITH EATING AND LIVING HEALTHY

Aside from the aforementioned, two other issues that people encounter when it comes to eating healthier and living healthier lives is the lack of: TIME AND THE COST OF HEALTHY FOOD.

Fact is, healthy food tends to be more expensive. If you do a quick browse at the grocery store, you'll see that the nuts, oats, and other similar food varieties cost more than your average take out. The reality is not everyone can afford it—but there are ways around this. So don't give up on eating healthy just yet!

Next, we have the issue of time which many people seem to lack these days. In particular, students and people who work 9 to 5 might find it difficult to sustain a healthy lifestyle. It's always more convenient to just get take out and eat whilst you're studying or working at home. It's easier, but it is doing more harm than good to your body. You're just not seeing the effects YET. But, fret not. I shall help you find ways to incorporate healthier routines into your life as well.

The thing is, we're trying to achieve holistic health and the only way we're going to succeed in it is if you find balance in your life. Of course, this isn't an overnight thing. You will have to put in effort and apply everything you learn through this book. What I ask of you now is to keep an open mind and to develop a sense of discipline, especially when it comes to taking care of yourself. As people, we always have excuses to avoid doing things that are the slightest bit difficult—something that's outside of our comfort zones. This will be one of those things, but it will pay off and you will benefit greatly from it.

Remember, it is your health and the quality of your life hanging at the balance. Ask yourself if you want to go for wants convenient yet unhealthy or if you want to live healthier by accommodating certain changes that are outside of your comfort zone.

The choice is always up to you.

THAT SAID, LET ME HELP YOU OUT. HERE'S WHAT I CAN TEACH YOU.

With this bootcamp I aim to provide and teach you a step by step method towards weight loss. Whilst you'll learn new things about weight loss, I have also broken down all that information to make sure that each one can be easily understood. This is important— the more you understand what you're doing, the better you will be at following it.

I will also provide you with different assignments and worksheets, making sure that you apply everything that you have learned in real life.

This is A FLUFF-FREE guide and my aim is to dispel any misconceptions and myths about nutrition that you may have picked up throughout your own diet journey. You will be provided with ample information to help you move forward and progress when it comes to your weight loss goals.

I will also help you learn more about the mental side to weight loss —how our habits and mindset influence our weight loss journey. I will help you understand how losing weight isn't just a matter of restricting your food intake or incorporating more physical activity. It is also about becoming more disciplined, developing better habits, and setting up systems that support your goals.

I have also incorporated different concepts from Eastern alternative medicine, which includes TCM or traditional Chinese medicine. Through this course, you will learn how to reconcile those concepts with ones from western nutrition. The idea is that our mind and thoughts are both important towards our overall well-being and weight loss. This is something that most diet programs don't even discuss. For example, were you aware that each time you get angry, you are also hurting your liver? Simple as that may seem, it can have multiple health-related side effects that you must be mindful of.

RECOGNIZE YOUR CORE MOTIVATORS.

When it comes to starting any sort of project or endeavor, it pays to reflect on why you're doing it in the first place. Take a piece of paper and answer the following:

Why do you care about weight loss?

Why do you want to do it?

What do you want to achieve?

Don't rush when answering this. In fully understanding your purpose, you'll find both direction and motivation. This motivator is important; think of it as the northstar during your journey. It will keep you going and it will guide you as well.

Now, remember that there's no right or wrong answer to these questions. There's no such thing as a shallow or vain goal. If you want to lose weight because you want to look more attractive, then that's a completely valid reason. If you're doing it to fit into a dress or to look great for a special event, those are valid reasons too. However, it is likely that your reasons go much deeper than the above examples—people who are serious about losing weight often do so because they want to create changes in their life. They want to improve their health.

Perhaps you're tired of feeling lethargic all the time. You might be a parent who wants to do everything for their children, but often find that you lack the energy to do so. After all, being able to keep up with your kids is important— but you won't be able to do that if your health is on the decline. Maybe that's part of your worry as well; that you're wasting resources on prescription medicines for your condition instead of using it for your family. You no longer want to miss out on vacations because you're always troubled by health insurance issues.

At the end of the day, want everyone wants is to be healthy— to be able to do all the things you want to and enjoy life without struggling with pain and other physical issues brought on by your weight issues.

LET'S TALK HOLISTIC HEALTH.

When we talk of holistic health, this refers to your overall well-being and not just one aspect of it such as weight loss. This will be the core of our course— the thing that will help trigger your weight loss. Basically, this means that your weight loss will be a direct and natural result of improving your health.

It's limiting to think of weight loss as merely losing fat in different areas of your body, without really considering as to how the act of achieving that affects your health. For example, if you focus too much on calorie counting and starvation diets, you will get results but at the cost of your health. It is unnatural and you will be causing more harm than good if you continue it. Remember, just because you're getting the results you want from a diet, it doesn't mean that you're doing things right.

Holistic health brings together the mind and body. It will enable you to change what you think about food, helping you understand that it is something that can directly affect your life. More than just something to fill your stomach with or something that you can use to pass the time, the food you consume can influence your mental and physical health.

It's all about choosing to eat healthier food, knowing that doing so can help you eliminate different health issues—including mood swings, low energy, and even chronic inflammation. Weight loss is just the cherry on top of that cake. You will learn that consuming good food is the basis for preventing these conditions from happening or reoccurring.

However, people aren't given this information. Have you ever tried going to the doctor's only to be provided with the same details you can find on Google? Basic things that don't really touch on the depth of the subject; things such as proper nutrition and obesity is a consequence of food addiction rather than just a result of consuming fatty food? Even in schools, I have observed that kids these days are only provided with the basics and often outdated ideas. There's a proliferation of incorrect advice online too—no wonder people feel so lost!

Then you have the problem with healthcare and how it can be so expensive that people don't even consider it an option. I say this from experience, back when I didn't know how healthcare worked and ended with a 500 dollar charge for a simple ear cleaning procedure. These doctors and nurses don't really discuss the finer details with patients. Instead, they bombard you with unnecessary information, stuff that the average man won't really understand. By the time you're through with the procedure you're getting, you might end up a few hundred dollars poorer.

GET YOUR MONEY'S WORTH.

That's the very thing this book aims to eliminate. You no longer have to wade through an ocean of information just to find the important bits. I'm giving you an easy-to-follow guide containing only the essentials that'll take you from point A to point Z when it comes to becoming healthier and losing weight. The only thing I request of you is that you really absorb the lessons and participate in it actively.

There will be different modules breaking down the information further, as well as assignments you must complete. If need be, repeat each one multiple times until you feel as if you've done enough. Remember, the goal here isn't speed—there's no need to rush through the course. What's important is that you're able to apply each new knowledge properly as you progress in your journey.

Think of this program as a giant project meant to change your life. Each module I'll be presenting you with is actionable and will produce real world results.

Let's jump right into it, shall we?

TERRIBLE 3'S: WEIGHT LOSS MISCONCEPTIONS YOU NEED TO UNLEARN

Previously, I provided you with a general overview of what the program is about. This time, we'll be tackling the 3 key weight loss misconceptions that most people have. I find that it's of importance to clear these up so that you can make better and more informed decisions when it comes to your weight loss journey.

It's Only Cosmetic

Fact: A lot of people want to lose weight because they believe that it will improve their external appearance. However, having this kind of mindset can also lead to the belief that weight loss is purely a cosmetic issue—one that is separate from other health factors that directly affect it.

For example, weight gain also serves as a sign that there's an imbalance in your overall health. It is linked to a number of chronic health issues and is known as the leading cause of it as well. Current estimates show that within the next twenty years or so, about 16 to 18% of all health care costs would be attributed to health issues caused by obesity. The cost of excessive weight is even outpacing cancer.

Look, these figures are not meant to scare you. Rather, I am merely painting a clearer picture for you—so you'll be able to understand that weight loss isn't a singular problem with a singular cause. You must first improve your lifestyle and focus on holistic health if you really want big changes to happen. You will feel better, not just physically, but mentally as well. Besides, with the exponentially rising healthcare costs in the USA, very few people can really afford to get sick. Imagine not being able to work, despite really wanting to, simply because your body's no longer fit for it. That's bound to take its toll on you, causing further issues.

So why let it get to that point, right?

Eating Less and Counting Calories

This is one of the most prevalent misconceptions about weight loss, something that you might even be following without realizing that you're doing it wrong. If you're unfamiliar with it, though, calorie counting works like this: you keep track of the calories you consume with every meal, then try to burn off more than that number during exercise at the end of the day. You give yourself a limit and try your best to not go beyond that number. Sounds pretty easy, right? It should be, if you're able to keep track of your calories throughout the day.

Then you add the physical activity, believing that by doing exercise for 30 minutes to an hour each day, you can make sure that your calorie count will not exceed the limit you have set. Say, running for half an hour on the treadmill to burn the excess away, only to realize after a few days that there are no real results from doing so. Instead, you're actually gaining a bit of weight—WHY? Well, that's because exercise does not do much for weight loss in comparison to eating right. This is one of the biggest misconceptions that people believe in. Whilst exercise is crucial for your overall health, pushing yourself to the brink of exhaustion during workouts will not be able to effectively lower your weight.

We'll get into more detail about that later, for now we shall be focusing on the issue of calorie counting.

So, what are you doing wrong? The process of what I call "calorie accounting" does not take into consideration the fact that not all calories are made equal. For example, if you consume 1000 calories per day that's derived from junk food, you're not getting proper nutrition and might even begin to feel physically sick. But if you're getting calories from proper food, not only are you nourishing your body, you're also providing it with fuel.

Then there's this thing with food accounting and how it trains your brain into prioritizing quantity instead of quality. Remember that it is never about eating the right amount of food (though, moderation is still key), but rather you must consider the kind of food you consume on a daily basis. Understanding the difference between quality food and the ones you should avoid can bring about drastic changes. More on that later.

WEIGHT LOSS IS IMPOSSIBLE

Lastly, we have this. Many people seem to believe that the whole process is impossible—which is quite understandable. It is likely that you and so many others have already tried different methods throughout the years, including reading different books and trying your best to squeeze in exercise even after a long day. This is especially so for people who have to take care kids along with other responsibilities—it almost feels as if there isn't enough time in a day to get everything done.

Nevertheless, most would start off strong in the beginning. However, once the initial excitement dies and the first month has passed, you find yourself slowing down until everything feels impossibly hard. Then comes the frustration and stress, which can sometimes to lead to cravings. More often than not, people seek out something fried or savory, even something sweet, whenever they feel stressed. Maintaining self-control and keeping oneself from being lazy is hard. Look, I've been in the same place before and empathize with using food as a crutch for sadness. For me, it was desserts and stress is a major trigger for my cravings.

But that's just one of the many challenges people face when it comes to trying to be healthier and lose weight. There's also the fact that, on a daily basis, we have so many things going on. Whether that be for school, work, or home related. This begs the question, how do we find the time to take care of ourselves better? I will address all of that and more, as we continue on. For now, I want you to understand that the process and your goals are not impossible to achieve. The tools are readily available and you have this step by step guide to help you overcome difficulties. Now, you just need to have the right mindset for it.

Think of the process as something similar to baking a cake for the first time. You already have all of the ingredients, but will that be enough for you to do it successfully? Will you even attempt it? Now, imagine someone providing you with a clear, step by step recipe; things just got a lot easier, right? Only then will you feel more confident and motivated to actually get started. That is what I aim to achieve with this program, to provide you with the steps so you feel more confident with going through the process. That's me holding your hand and guiding you towards achieving your health and weight loss goals.

Is weight loss impossible? Not anymore!

Another point I want to make is this: After passing a certain threshold, you will find that the process of being healthy and losing weight begins to get easier. This is usually a consequence of switching to healthier food—where your body starts to adapt to the changes and any cravings you have for junk food begins to decrease until they disappear. What happens is a snow ball effect. Based on my experience, after just a few weeks of switching to eating healthier, I could no longer handle eating junk foods such as chips and packaged noodles. In fact, after eating them, I began to have symptoms such as fatigue, nausea, and even depression!

The point is this: Getting to this stage will be challenging, but once you manage to get there, things do get easier. Just keep the hope and stay disciplined!

A RECAP: Before we close this phase of the program, let's recap the lessons you've been given thus far:

Misconception 1: Weight gain is purely cosmetic. Remember, it is a symptom or a sigh that things are not right in your body.

Misconception 2: Losing weight can be achieved by simply counting calories and exercising. Fact is, exercise does little when it comes to helping you lose weight, but it is essential for overall health.

Misconception 3: Losing weight is not impossible, no matter how big you are right now. All the tools you need is inside you, you simply have to do things one step at time with discipline.

3 ESSENTIAL KEYS TO WEIGHT LOSS

Whenever we think of weight loss or the process of accomplishing it, most of the time our minds go to one or all of the following: slaving for hours at the gym, struggling with saying NO to the food we enjoy, and some form of torture that usually turns people away from it before even getting started. Sounds about, right? Well, contrary to all of the aforementioned, the 3 core concepts is far from being painful—in fact, you might be surprised at what they actually are.

MASTERING THE MIND.

Before you work on your body, you must first work and master your mind. In fact, 80% of holistic weight loss largely resides in the mind. What this means is that you'll need to master your thoughts and your habits, destroying your bad relationship with food that's ultimately damaging your health. After, you must also train your mind in order to build and maintain new and much better habits that will help sustain holistic health.

How to begin? Start by implementing a number of small habits slowly but surely. It is said that it takes about 30 days for a habit to really stick— this may not seem like much, but if you're making changes then it can feel like an insurmountable challenge. However, it is NOT IMPOSSIBLE. Start small and work your way up. For example:

Dealing with stress properly. By now, I hope you already see the connection between our mental well-being and weight gain. Bad emotions, stress, anger—all these things contribute to our weight gain whether that be directly or indirectly. So, what better place to start than there? In breaking down and understanding stress better, you should be able to move on to eliminating bad habits —such as relying on bad food to get through your days, to feel something, and so on.

RELEARNING NUTRITION.

Next, you need to relearn and update what you know about basic nutrition. As I have emphasized early on, there is plenty of myths surrounding weight loss, fats, and what really causes weight gain. In having ample knowledge about nutrition, you build up a strong foundation for creating a healthier lifestyle. You'll have the information you need for making better choices when shopping and a better understanding of the right kind of food for your body.

All of which are important if you really want to make healthy changes and sustain it throughout your life.

MAINTAINING A SYSTEM.

Lastly, it is important for you to create a system that would aid you in continuously implementing all the step by step strategies I'll be providing you with. This includes going through with a personal meal plan and maintaining all of the new habits you have developed.

SIMPLE STRATEGIES FOR BETTER SLEEP

Physical and mental, you must remember this when it comes to holistic health. The bridge between the two is sleep and as such, it is a very important aspect of holistic weight loss. As we have discussed, everything is connected. In this case, if you don't get enough sleep, you can end up with mood swings and become irritable. Your performance will also suffer and your stress will continue to mount—all of that leads to an increase in your craving for snacks which will result in weight gain.

Did you know that a lack of sleep can increase your likelihood of early death—especially one that's been caused by cardiovascular issues? Sleep allows your mind and body to heal, if you're not getting enough of it then you're damaging your body more and more without giving it a chance to recover.

Another thing to keep in mind is the fact that all biology in this world follows the natural rhythm of our planet. As humans, we are no exception to this. Our different bodily processes follow a similar pattern, including our nervous system, immune system, and hormones. If this pattern gets disrupted, it causes imbalances and other issues in our body. Just think back to all the times you have gotten ill after days of not being able to sleep properly. Didn't you feel completely drained of energy and your thoughts absolutely foggy? Keep in mind you circadian rhythm.

Now, not everyone has been blessed with the ability to get a peaceful night's sleep. Some of us have trouble because of inherent issues and illnesses. Some, some struggle because they carry the stresses of the day into bed with them. No matter the reason, it is important that you find a way to get enough sleep at proper times. Here are some tips you could try:

Melatonin is fine to use, but make sure you only gradually increase its use. Talk to an expert about this or someone who has experience using it. The more you know and understand about it, the better. For younger folks, particularly the teenagers, you'll need to take it earlier than most. For example, if you want to fall asleep by 10, you should take it by 7.

Make sure your room is conducive to sleeping. This means that it should be dark and that you have turned off all blue light devices an hour before hitting the sack. Temperatures should be comfortable as well.

Always set a predictable sleep time for yourself. An hour before, you should do your best to de-stress. Try a bit of meditation before going to bed. Also, make sure that you don't drink coffee or eat anything within that hour. Doing so can easily disrupt your sleep pattern.

A good diet is also key to better sleep. When it comes to regulating circadian rhythms, one of the best vitamins to take as supplement would be vitamin D.

THE TRUTH BEHIND EXERCISE AND WHY YOU ONLY NEED LITTLE OF IT

Now we have reached the point where we must clear up one of the biggest misconceptions when it comes to weight loss. Plenty of people seem to believe that in order to lose weight, doing a lot of exercise is all they need. This is why you'll often find people running on the treadmill for an hour straight, thinking that it would help them burn off the fat and shed pounds.

In fact, I have a friend who goes to gym everyday for about 2 hours for each session. However, despite months of doing so, very little has changed when it comes to his weight. Why? Because it's not exercise that sheds the pounds off—it's what you eat. It's your diet.

Look, I'm not trying to say that you should stop exercising. Of course not—physical activity is still very important for maintaining holistic health. But doing that alone will not help you lose weight. There are many benefits to exercising, however. This includes its effects as a mood booster, how it helps reduce blood sugar levels in the body, and lowers your likelihood of developing chronic diseases. It can also help heavy metals such as mercury and cadmium from your body through sweating.

If you're a beginner, here are my suggested exercise routines:

One of the best ways to get started is by doing moderate exercise —the idea here is that you shouldn't push yourself too hard, especially if this is your first time doing constant physical activity. Begin by doing exercises for 30 minutes a day, about 4 to 5 times each week. Running 5 miles vs. 3 miles has marginal benefit.

Another thing you should do is weight train for about 15 minutes, once or twice a week. You need not spend hours a day at the gym in order to stay healthy. Doing the minimum, but doing it regularly is more than enough maintenance.

WEEK 2:

YOUR BEHAVIOR AFFECTS WEIGHT LOSS AND WEIGHT GAIN—

Let's begin this phase by touching on some basics when it comes to human psychology and behavior. Previously, I discussed that weight is largely due to poor diet and choices—two things which are also dictated by habits and behavior. It doesn't matter how much information you manage to amass, all of that would go to nothing if you don't take action and actually apply it to your life.

This means that you must begin with your behavior, changing it to align with your fitness and weight loss goals. The same applies to any goals you have, really. Every mind works differently, so it is also important that you gain an understanding of how yours works. What motivates you? This, among other questions, will be answered in this module. I will teach you how to build better habits and make it stick—I will be giving you the necessary building blocks to get you started on your journey.

HUMAN BEHAVIOR AND ITS 3 FACES

Think of human behavior as having 3 different faces, each one essential to the whole. You will need to understand every aspect of it in order to make it work.

MOTIVATION

To put it simply, this is the WHY behind any person's behavior. Earlier, I gave you the task of writing down a list of your motivators—this is important because you have to recognize what fuels you and gets you to do something. More often than not, this is a thing that gives you pleasure, social acceptance, hope, and so on. It could also a type of fear. Perhaps you don't want to end up being sickly and not be able to do the things you want in life. Needless to say, motivation can be many different things—varying from one person to another.

For me, it was the fear of not being able to live the life I wanted. I was young and I had many dreams. I wanted to travel, I wanted to succeed, I wanted to someday have my own family, and I wanted to be healthy enough to experience all of that. The fear of not being able to made me develop better habits. It made me choose better food as well. Each time I felt like I was faltering in my journey or losing the will to continue, it is this fear that motivated me to push forward.

That said, there are also certain things you must know about the power of motivation. Firstly, know that it can help you get started but it will not be enough to sustain your journey. As I've mentioned, it is but a fuel—a catalyst—but you will have to adopt a system alongside it in order to keep going. That's where your habits come in. Simply relying on motivation and willpower is, in fact, a losing strategy. It doesn't matter what you've been told before, no one ever achieves anything if it's just these two powering them on.

Why? Because it's too much hard work and motivation can be a very fickle thing.

Think back to all the times you were fired up to get started; the first week of losing weight was amazing for you. You begin with so much motivation, so much fuel speeding you forward, only to lose it some time afterwards. This is also why so many people fail with their New Year's resolutions. The start of a new year always brings with it such good energy, the motivation to turn a new leaf and become a new person, but that only lasts a few weeks into it. If you're lucky, maybe a month or two.

Then, it is all but forgotten. Everyone's got their own excuse, but we don't really have time to talk about that, do we?

ABILITY

This refers to how easy it is to act out a certain type of behavior. Case in point: eating healthier. If you're someone who has responsibilities on top of other responsibilities, you will most likely have to prioritize which one comes first. I don't blame you for not always putting healthy eating first. When you're dealing with school or work, children, and other home-related tasks which leave you exhausted by the end of the day, cooking becomes the last thing you want to do.

So, I understand why you might reach for take-out food more often than not. It is so convenient, after all. You need not think about which ingredients to buy and actually go through the motions of preparing the food you want. That said, I understand the situation but it does not mean that I condone it and neither should you. Yes, it's not easy—but I will help you find a way.

TRIGGER

This is the thing that makes you act. One of the most common examples of which can be found on social media. If you use websites such as Facebook, Pinterest, and other similar platforms, then you'll know exactly what I'm referring to. Perhaps you saw an inspiring story about how someone managed to lose weight after years of failure; it could have gotten you thinking and looking at your situation more.

Think of this is a friendly nudge that gets you to think and then do the behavior.

It doesn't even have to be big. Maybe it's a dress on Pinterest that you really liked and want to be able to fit into. Perhaps it's a content creator on YouTube who has inspired you to live a more mindful, healthier life. We are often faced with these triggers, but very few really manage to nudge us into action.

THE BEHAVIOR EQUATION.

In order for a particular behavior to occur, all three of its components must align. This is what I refer to as the behavior equation. To paint a clearer picture, imagine this:

You are browsing your favorite social media one day, looking through your favorite accounts, or reading your favorite bloggers, when something catches your attention. Perhaps it's someone putting together an organic recipe book to help people with eating cleaner and healthier. You purchase it immediately, knowing that this is something you've been wanting to try. You are very motivated, even following through with the recipes for the first week.

However, things begin to slowly take a nose dive come the second week. You are still motivated, by bogged down by your ability to make it happen. Perhaps, you don't have enough time to purchase the ingredients you need, maybe the ingredients are a bit too pricy for what's left of your budget, or maybe you're around people who always eat a certain type of food—the kind that's bad for you. There's a lot of other factors that can hinder you and create an imbalance in the behavior equation.

Of course, this leads to non-action on your part. The very thing we're seeking to avoid.

Here's an assignment for you:

BEHAVIOR	MOTIVATION	ABILITY	TRIGGER

Write down a behavior that you want to develop. It could be anything from "eating healthier, sleeping better, avoiding stress-eating, and so on."

List down your motivations.

Next to that, write down the things that you are capable of doing and those that might be hindering you from completing the action.

Finally, write down triggers that you encounter that nudge you towards taking action or inaction.

GOAL: This should help you recognize some of the behavioral issues you might have, the things hindering you from successfully integrating healthier habits into your life. It would be good to do this assignment with an honest heart and open mind. Recognizing your flaws isn't a bad thing, in fact, it can help propel you forward without fear.

THE ANATOMY OF HABITS: 3 CORE FACTORS

Before we move forward, let's be clear about this: habits are different from behaviors. Your behavior towards something is typically a one-time thing—bottomline is, it can change at any given time. Habits, on the other hand, are a repeating series of behaviors. It isn't always as easy to change. Picture this:

You're stressed out after a long day of working and handling household matters. So stressed that you begin craving food. The bag of salty and greasy chips in the pantry is the first thing that comes to mind. Now, your behavior could go two different ways. One, you go and grab the chips. Or two, you opt to make yourself an easy banana smoothie instead to help distress. Your motivation, ability, and trigger determines which option you go for.

Habit, on the other hand, will put you on autopilot and go for the option you ALWAYS choose. In this case, it is likely that you'll grab the bag of chips, finish it off, and call it a night. The whole act is subconscious, there's no real consideration to it and you're only after an immediate reward. I'm certain we have all experienced this—especially when it comes to dealing with our cravings.

We all know how difficult dealing with food cravings can be. It is one of the major detriments people experience when trying to lose weight or simply trying to be healthy. Blame that on the years of us being taught to use food as a crutch. Eating a tub of ice cream whenever heartbroken? Shoving chips and other bad food into our mouth whenever stressed? Even media tends to glamorize this and people follow suit. But truth be told, this is nothing short of being an addiction. A very extreme and dangerous form of a habit.

In my case, I went through a period in my life where I felt like I was being bombarded by stress on the daily. Everything seemed to be going wrong or was on the verge of it. During this time, I was applying for university and had way too much piled onto my plate. There were hours upon hours of work to be done; from homework, application essays, social activities, and other responsibilities on top of all that.

I remember clearly how whenever I would get stuck on doing my applications, I would feel the urge to go out and grab some fast food. Stuff that I knew was bad, but I simply had no control over my cravings. It became a habit that felt impossible to quit—

that's when I understood the dangers of it. Once it has taken root, stopping it can be the most difficult thing to do. It takes enormous willpower and effort. Before I knew it, I had piled on the pounds.

HOW AND WHY DO HABITS DEVELOP?

According to a majority of research, many bad habits are a result of two things: STRESS AND BOREDOM. In a study done by York University, among others academic institutions, the two are actually closely linked. During times of stress, your pre-frontal cortex, which is the part of your brain responsible for your rationale thought, shuts off. This is when all consideration goes out the door and the brain only seeks reward. For our primitive ancestors, this was a form of survival. However, with resources at the ready, modern man doesn't have much need for this particular instinct.

Now, think about the bad habits that you have. Typically, these can be categorized into two different groups. For example, stress triggers certain habits that we have—this can be eating junk food as a form of distraction or it could also be biting your nails to get the tension out. The same can be said if you're bored, the mind immediately craves something to occupy it. This is something that many people can relate to, in fact, you might be feeling either stress or bored right now. Not to worry, I will teach you healthier ways of dealing with it.

THREE COMPONENTS OF A HABIT

Previously, we have learned the different components of behavior. Habits are composed of three different components as well, with behavior being among those. Why is it important to learn these things, you might ask? Whether you're starting or trying to quit something, understanding how something works really helps. The same goes if you're trying to change your bad habits to good ones; working on things right from the source will not only produce stronger results, it also teaches you what to avoid in the future.

After all, you wouldn't want repeats, right?

That said, let's get to the different components that comprise a habit.

BEHAVIOR

As we have established, behavior pertains to the act itself—the action we take in response to a situation. It's you driving out to get junkfood whenever you're stressed. It's your decision to while away boredom by snacking on some chips or quenching your thirst with a can of soda instead of water.

Now, it's time for an assignment.

STRESSOR	FOOD CRAVING	NOTES

Using the above list, write down some of your stressors or bad habits and the food craving associated with it. Whether that be drinking soda everyday or finishing an entire pack of chips whenever you're bored. It could also be that milk tea and boba addiction, something that you tend to have more than once every single day.

The goal here is to recognize the common stressors you have and if there's a way to reduce or eliminate them all together. In doing so, you should be able to reduce your craving for bad food as well. Make sure you observe any changes that happen along the way!

REWARD

Reward is basically a portion of the habit loop that happens after you do the action. To make that a bit clearer, indulging in a slice of your favorite cake after a very long day. Or your morning cup of coffee after you wake up, helping you feel more energized. All of these things make you feel great and satiated; because of that, your mind starts to think of these things as rewards. And what do we know about our mind?

It likes rewards.

It is important to note that every habit ends in a reward. Even the act of brushing your teeth comes with one—that would be the tingling, clean feeling it leaves in your mouth. Since rewards are positive, your brain remembers it and would want to repeat it over and over again. With enough repetition, it becomes a habit and becomes ingrained in your mind.

That said, it is also important that the food you're craving might not even be the actual reward. What this means is that, it only serves as a proxy or a coping mechanism—something that your brain instantly turns to because you're not really giving it other alternatives. Case in point: There was one time I wanted to test out if my burger cravings was the reward my brain wanted. After a long day at work, one that was particularly stressful, I opted to go for a walk instead of heading to my favorite burger place.

Within 15 minutes of my walk, I realized that I was no longer craving the burger.

Now, let's tackle another assignment. For this, our goal is to figure out what the actual reward is behind your food craving—basically, which cravings is driving your behavior. The rules are pretty simple. Do this over a span of a few days, maybe even a week. It is important that you don't rush it and that you don't change any of your ways.

HOW IT WORKS:

Go through your usual routine when it comes to the food cravings you have. Don't overthink it and don't change any of your actions.

Now, each time you experience a craving, switch up your behavior to something different. Try about 5 to 6 different alternatives. For example: Feel like going for a late night donut run? Change that to a few minutes of yoga instead. How about playing video games or watching some YouTube as an alternative? You can also opt to call a friend for a chat or if you really feel like eating, grab a healthier snack or make yourself a nice up of tea. You can even have coffee!

The point here is to experiment with a different action or behavior whenever your craving comes. You're bound to find something that your brain responds to. Trust me on this one.

That said, observe your own feelings each time you switch up your reward. After 15 minutes, are you still craving for the same thing? You can even take notes, this should help you better understand the reason behind your cravings. It could be that you're merely looking for a distraction—which was what happened in my case. All those times I craved a burger? My mind simply wanted to focus on something else other than my work worries.

As you continue with this assignment, make sure that you change your "rewards" to something far better and healthier. For example, instead of reaching for a soda or junk food, opt for coffee. If your mind responds to it—the reward it wanted was energy all along. If your cravings were satiated by a healthy meal that doesn't include all the greasy stuff you thought you were craving, the reward it wanted was to satisfy hunger. Be more mindful and observant, it helps a lot.

Remember, there's no timetable to this process. You might figure things out within a week, maybe you even need double that. The idea is to understand your cravings and the real reason behind it so take your time. You can use the template below for your notes:

BEHAVIOR	MOTIVATION	ABILITY	TRIGGER

TRIGGER

As the name suggests, this is the thing that gives your brain the cue for craving. For most people, the common trigger is stress. However, this isn't the only one. Know that there are also different categories for triggers:

Environment

First up, we have the location or environment you're in. we often pay very little attention to it, but this is actually one of the most powerful triggers people are faced with. You may not even think that something is a trigger because you're so used to it.

Case in point: An open pantry in the office or a plate of treats, such as cookies and candies, that's free for anyone's taking. If you see it there, knowing that it's alright for you to take some, you're likely to be compelled to do just that—even if you weren't even thinking about the snacks beforehand. Sound familiar? The same goes for when you're at home.

Going back to motivation, ability, and trigger--- applied in this situation, your location and environment certainly makes your ability to do the behavior much easier (it's right in front of you, after all), but it also acts as a trigger at the same time. Talk about a double punch! Following that logic, you can use this equation to create good changes in your life as well.

For example: Do you want to start drinking more water throughout the day? Place a bottle or a cup by your countertop and remove all the soda in your home. You'll likely reach for that water because you'll be reminded to every time you see it. Want to watch less TV? Hide the remote, cover your TV, or if you're looking for something more drastic—you can even opt to hide the TV itself. Only do this if you live alone or have the permission of your housemates, of course.

It might seem like overreacting to some, but trust me, you have to do what is needed in order to change your bad habits. If that is what'll do it—by all means, go for it.

Time

Next, we have time. This isn't about timing—think daily rituals that happen at a specific time of day. For example, everyone has a morning ritual that they follow. Some people would make coffee straight away upon waking up and only after that do they wash their face, brush their teeth, etc. Because this is something that we do every single day without fail, the act becomes automatic. We hardly even think about what step to take next, we just follow our usual pattern.

Emotional State

This involves your feelings such as boredom, sadness, stress, heartbreak, even positive ones such as joy. These can all be triggers, as we've emphasized early on. Some people feel the need to "drown their misery" in food, whilst there are also those who celebrate by overindulging. Note that not every emotional trigger is negative, we just have to be observation of our own behavior and habits.

The People Around Us

Much like our environment, we hardly pay attention to the influence that people have on us. The presence of our friends, family, and other acquaintances can actually trigger us to do something. If you suddenly meet a friend that you really like, that instance can trigger a certain behavior on your part.

There is a saying that goes, "You are the average of your five closest friends" and if we apply this to health, it make sense. In fact, there's a study that backs this up. The New England Journal of Medicine published a study that points out the fact that being friends with someone who is obese can increase your own risk of obesity by 57%. Now, this isn't to say that you shouldn't be friends with anyone who is overweight—the point is that, you can get influenced by some of their habits unless you're mindful.

The Action that Precedes Your Craving

What is this referring to exactly? Well, think of it this way. When you hear that familiar alert from your iPhone, you automatically feel a desire to check it whatever you might be doing at the moment. The same goes for food. Let's say you've settled down for the evening to watch a movie or play your favorite video game, the mere act of doing so can trigger a craving for the usual snacks that you have and make you feel as if the experience is "incomplete" if you don't get it.

BREAKING THE BAD: KICKING YOUR OLD HABITS TO THE CURB

Previously, we have discussed the different components that comprise a habit. To recap, this is the trigger, which cues the behavior, which then gives you the reward. We've also done a few assignments meant to help you identify your personal bad habits, its triggers, and the real reward behind it. To further drive the point home, I'll tell you my own experience:

For me, I identified my trigger, which was stress from essays and applications—this usually happens late at night, around 10pm. This then triggered me to go out to get my favorite junk foods such as donuts and milk tea. At first, I wasn't really paying attention to this particular habit forming, but when I began gaining weight? I started to be more mindful.

Through observation and some trial and error, I was able to discover that the real reward behind this craving was distraction. My brain wanted a pause from all the studying and mounting stress. This was satisfied by the act of getting junk food.

The great thing about finally understanding your bad habits is that you can now begin to break them. You must have heard or read about many different ways of doing this—you might have even tried a few for self-improvement but it is likely that your success was minimal. After all, you're still reading this and looking for answers. Before we get to the actual process of breaking the habit, let's tackle some of the misconceptions associated with it first.

THE BIGGEST MISCONCEPTION ABOUT BREAKING A BAD HABIT

It's not about suppressing your habit—sure, that's going to work a few times, but you're not exactly tackling the problem at its root. This is important for you to understand because this is where so many fail when it comes to this process. Why? Because the mind works this way: The more you see something, the more you end up thinking about it. Merely thinking about something can become a trigger for a craving—I'm sure you're familiar with this.

Think about the times you had a craving and you tried to suppress it through distraction. However, the thought of it is persistent and in the end, it becomes uncontrollable so you end up succumbing to it. This can apply to other things besides junk food. But, what does it mean for you then? Well, it points to a key factor in breaking a habit effectively: Substituting a new, better action for your previously bad habit.

A STEP BY STEP GUIDE TO BREAKING A BAD HABIT:

Going back to our previous lesson, we've talked about how habits occur because of three different components. Following that logic, we can break a bad food habit by eliminating one of those components—which will lead to the entire link breaking down in consequence.

First, let's tackle behavior. The simple idea here is to replace your bad behavior with a better one. Basically, it goes like this: If you like soda, but know that it is bad for you and want to drink more water instead, act on the craving differently when it happens. The process, of course, requires constant practice. Since we all know that resistance is futile, what you can do is give into the behavior--- but eliminate the bad aspect of it. Picture this:

Back when I was struggling with this step, I realized that my cravings were actually serving as mere distractions from my bouts with stress. What I did, instead of running out to buy junk food like I usually would, is I changed the action associated with the cravings. I still went out, but I went for a quick jog rather than going to the convenience store or my favorite fast food. Whenever running wasn't an option, I went for a walk or got on the phone with friend, to chat and catch up. This effectively "killed" my cravings and I was able to distract myself in a healthy, more productive way.

Looking for suggestions on what you can do instead of eating bad food? Consult the list below whenever you run out of ideas:

Organize your bookshelf (or just your shelf in general).

Bust out the vacuum cleaner and clean your room or the entire house.

Do simple breathing exercises. If you're stressed, this is helpful for clearing out your mind.

Grab a book, one that you enjoy, and start reading.

You can also opt to do simple watercolor drawings. You need not be any good at it, but art can be very therapeutic and helpful for keeping stress at bay.

Knitting and crocheting! Because this requires a certain degree of focus, these should be very effective for taking your mind off of your persistent cravings.

Watch and inspiring YouTube video or listen to a related podcast.

If you're not too keen on activities, you can also substitute your bad food habit with healthier ones. This means switching out the junk food for better options. Below are a few examples that don't require any prep or cooking. Quick fixes for sudden cravings!

Want chips? Switch it up and choose for different nuts instead. There are also healthier options for chips, but these might be a little pricy and some are only sold in specific stores. Nuts are easily accessible, they taste good, are healthy, and quite affordable as well.

Looking for sweets? It would be very easy to just grab another chocolate bar or a few pieces of candy, but you can also satisfy your craving with a teaspoon of organic honey. It's great for your throat and has antioxidant properties as well.

Let's pause for a moment—now, think about the food that you tend to crave for the most. I'm sure you'll find it hard to really think about a healthier alternative for it, but that's what the second "attack" is for.

Next, we have the trigger. Going back to our soda analogy. If soda is one of your favorites, thus making it hard for you to just find an alternative for it, then what must be done is to get rid of any cues that make it easy for you to drink it. Basically: THROW THAT SODA AWAY. If you'd rather not waste it, however, give it to someone who only has it ever so often.

Once you've gotten rid of it, now's the time to replace it with a POSITIVE trigger. Where your soda used to be, place water or infused water in its spot. In fact, if you really want to push yourself towards drinking more water, place water bottles where you can EASILY access it. Think: nightstand, by the couch, on your work desk, and so on. If your bad food habit tends to happen at a particular time—in my case, I always seem to crave fast food right around midnight whenever I'm working—this calls for scheduling new actions into your life.

Again, this is all about taking all the necessary measures towards making big changes happen. If you have to schedule your new habit with an alarm, DO IT! Make it a daily thing and make sure you do the alternate behavior each time. PRO TIP: Use a song that you really like for your alarm. This will immediately put you in a good mood AND associate positive feelings with the alternate behavior you're trying to develop. Doing this should make it easier for your brain to adjust as well.

Lastly, it's time we handled the reward—quite possibly, the hardest one to tackle.

Because the reward makes you feel good and satiates your craving, what you must do is reverse the effect it gives you. This is particularly difficult, of course, but one thing that can help is writing down the ill effects that you feel after you drink the soda. Whether that be a stomachache, yellow or weak teeth, bad skin, and so on, list it down and stick it on your fridge where you can easily see just before you grab another can.

Alternatively, you can also create a habit calendar or tracker. Stick this on your fridge and each time you go for water instead of soda, stick a star on that calendar or simply make a mark on it. The idea here is that you're switching the reward you get from the soda to something that gives you an equally positive feeling--- every mark on that calendar means you're succeeding and progressing. There's no greater feeling than that.

*We will discuss the habit calendar / tracker later on to make sure you get the idea.

What you need to remember, is that breaking a bad food habit or any bad habit for that matter, will require some trial and error. If you fail at first, that doesn't mean you have failed completely and should give up no. On the contrary, take that failure as your first lesson and then try something else. Make sure you write down your observations and know that even small progresses count.

BUILDING GOOD HABITS AND MAKING THEM STICK

After you're done breaking all the bad habits, it's time you put in place some new and BETTER ones. Now, mindfully building a habit will not be as easy as developing one on auto-pilot. That said, you are already armed with knowledge from the previous lessons so you have a good idea about what a habit is. To quickly recap, habits are composed of three parts—very much like a chain. You have your behavior, your trigger, and your reward. To break them, attack and eliminate one so that the chain falls apart.

To build a good chain, tackle your behavior first. Habits are like behaviors on steroids so it only goes that you will need to work with the 3 different components of behavior in order to make change happen. Those three are: motivation, ability, and trigger.

Let's start with motivation since this tends to be the most problematic for people. I understand how difficult it can be trying to maintain this; how one moment you're feeling ready to lose weight and change your unhealthy eating habits, only to lose that energy the following day. Needless to say, motivation can be very fickle and relying on it in order to progress isn't always the best idea. It's good to find motivation in the beginning, but you're better off working with things you have more control over.

That brings us to triggers. How do you make sure that there is always some form of trigger that'll help cue your new habit? For example, what if you want to incorporate more vegetables into your current diet? Well, a good tip here is to utilize your already existing habit. Think about some that you have every single day, something like brushing your teeth every morning or doing stretches as soon as you get out of bed. For parents, maybe the first thing you do upon waking up is checking on your children then checking your email.

Around lunch time, perhaps you're the type to walk around after eating or maybe you always find yourself browsing for a new book just before lunchtime is through. When you get home at night, the first thing you do is sit down with your children for a fun chat or perhaps you feed the pets as a family routine. What I'm getting at is there will always be those habits that are deeply rooted in our lives, ones that do us no harm, and have simply become part of our everyday. It would only be logical to use these as a trigger for developing new ones, right? This is what's referred to as HABIT LINKING or HABIT STACKING—both mean the same thing.

It's tying a new habit into your current existing one in order to further the process.

Lastly, we have ability. As humans, it is pretty much in our nature to prefer the easy route and this is what I plan on helping you with. How can we make sure that you have the best possible ability for your new behavior? Well, the simple answer is this: We make it very easy for you to do the behavior THEN it into an already existing habit. So, what happens is you complete your existing habit then immediately after, you take one baby step into that new habit you're trying to build. Pat yourself on the back even for small successes. Trust me, you will feel more motivated to complete it each and every time.

Let's break this down into a simple formula: After I __________. I will _________.

Basically:

After I put the kids to sleep, I will __________.

After I come home from work, I will _________.

After I help the kids with homework, I will ___.

After I brush my teeth, I will _________.

Simple, right?

Now, onto an example you can follow.

Let's say that you want to build the habit of drinking 8 cups of water a day. The first thing you need to do is select a habit that you already do every single day. In my case, I always stretch every morning after the alarm goes off. After this, I pretty much spend a few minutes sat on my bed before putting on my socks. This leaves a few minutes wherein I'm not really doing much so this is a good place to incorporate my first steps into building the habit.

On day 1, I'll place a shot glass of water next to my bed. I'm using a shot glass because it's tiny and is very, very easy to drink. I don't even have to think about it. Repeat this for the next few days, perhaps for a week before changing that shot glass to a full cup. You can even opt to place a bottle of water next to your bed and make sure you take that bottle and hold it in your hand within a few moments after waking up. It might sound silly, but repeat this every single day and it's bound to stick. Eventually, you can even link this new water drinking behavior to your other existing habits--- perhaps before each meal, perhaps before your morning coffee.

RECAP: 5 STEPS TO BUILDING GOOD HABITS

Step one: Select an existing habit. Make sure they aren't vague. The more concrete it is, the better.

Step two: Start with small steps. Perform this right after your existing habit.

Step three: Always celebrate after performing the habit. This will motivate you and associate the act with a positive feeling. Your brain will love this.

Step four: Repeat this multiple times throughout the day. Continue it for 5 days to a week. Keep the ball rolling and you'll find that it's slowly becoming natural to you.

HABIT TRACKING

Breaking and building new habits aren't the only things you need to do. There's a final step that would help make sure your new habits are maintained for the long term—that is habit tracking.

Building habits can be a long-term process that takes a lot of experimentation. We've established that motivation cannot necessarily sustain it, but motivation can help you keep going. It can help keep you focused on your goal and provide you with a type of reward that satisfied your mind. This is where tracking enters the picture, it will help you keep track of your progress and provides the feedback you need to see that you're making the right moves.

Think of it as a more visual representation of what you know and feel. Yes, you feel lighter and healthier, bit there will be times when you'll require something more concrete. Especially those days when you might feel as if you have reached a plateau with your progress—something that can eventually happen, even I have experienced this. A tracker will show you your weight loss journey, just how much you have progressed, and the results of your hard work. It's no different from a professional athelete tracking their improvement.

Now, this tracker need not be fancy but it would be great if you're able to see it easily everyday. Put it on the fridge door or that of your closet, then place a mark each day you're able to progress. Below is a weekly example, but you can always adjust it to a monthly version.

HABITS	MON	TUE	WED	THURS	FRI	SAT	SUN
Weight	68						66
Sculpt	★			★		★	
Vegetables	★	★	★	★	★	★	★
More H20	★	★	★	★	★	★	★
No sugar			★	★	★		★
Running	★	★		★	★	★	
Yoga		★		★		★	

Along with this chart, you can also create a small visual board with quotes and sayings that help keep you inspired. You can put up photos of your children beside it and make them your motivation for getting healthier. Anything that will help keep your mindset positive will be very helpful towards your progress.

I'm sure you're asking— It's just a chart, will it actually work? The answer is YES. This tracker doesn't just keep tabs on your progress, it also serves as a reminder for you to act. If the growing trend of habit tracking apps becoming even more widespread is any indication, the method really helps. Plenty has been written about the modern man's obsession with what's referred to as "the quantified self". We all keep logs of every part of our daily lives, though we do so in different ways. There's bullet journals, lists, photo diaries, food logs, etc.

Habit formation trackers work in a similar manner. These things put the spotlight on our lives, distilling into actual data that we can study. With this data, we will be able to see what we need to improve on, what we need to do less, and how we can lead more balanced life. Basically, it propels us towards our ideal self; whether that be personality-wise, lifestyle-wise, and in you case, health-wise. With the help of these trackers, you can become that person you want—someone who eats healthily, exercises everyday, and is mentally-balanced despite everyday challenges.

It also makes your more mindful of what you do every single day, making sure that you do not slip into auto-pilot mode and your old bad habits as well. As we have continuously emphasized, the process of losing weight is mostly mental. It requires that you become more aware and give more consideration to what you do every single day with regards to your health. Habit trackers will help you do exactly that.

THE REWARD CONNECTION

Think of it this way, wouldn't it be nice to see those checkmarks all lined up for every single day you manage to succeed? The positive feelings that seeing the tracker gives you is registered by your brain, associating the act with something good. Now, imagine if it's posted on your pantry or the fridge—the next time you go and grab food that you know isn't good for you, you'll immediately think twice about continuing. Do you really want to ruin your streak?

Aside from that, it is also a reward for those around you. If you live with family or have one of your own, you can get them involved in the process and enjoy the satisfaction that comes with progressing with each day that comes.

All of that aside, I also want you to be kind to yourself whenever you have off days. Yes, we all want to do great and keep up the streak, but humans are prone to making mistakes as well. This is normal and you should not berate yourself if you happen to fail on certain days. What you can do, instead, is meditate on what led to your slip-up and if there's anything you can do to avoid it happening a second time.

WEEK 3:

THE SECRET TO STRESS MANAGEMENT—

The last module taught you plenty about building and creating better habits. It is important that you fully understand those concepts because they will serve as the building blocks that you'll need in order to achieve holistic weight loss. Make sure that you also practice that principles you were introduced; apply them to your life bit by bit. That's how we're going to sustain this process and your progress. This is no race, after all. Just pace yourself accordingly.

Now, for a quick recap:

BEHAVIOR is made up of 3 things: motivation, ability, and trigger. Each of these need to be higher than the activation threshold in order for the behavior to actually happen. We have also discussed what HABITS are, think behavior but on steroids. This is when the behavior happens without needing too much effort from you, basically an auto-pilot mode. Habits can also be good and bad—in the case of food, it usually is bad and must be changed.

So, what's that got to do with stress management?

As we've established, holistic health is key to weight loss. This includes eating healthy, living healthy, and tackling the weight problem right at its root which is a deeply mental one. Most overweight people tend to use food as an emotional crutch for whenever they feel stressed or depressed. They have a tendency to indulge in bad food, continuing the cycle until it severely affects their health. The trouble with stopping or changing is that this bad habit can become an addiction, something hardwired into their brains making it very difficult to make positive changes.

With that in mind, it only makes sense that we address stress in order to resolve the issue from its core.

Did you know that our emotions are linked to different organs in our body? This is according to traditional Chinese medicine where it is believed that everything which makes up a human being, the mind, the body, and the spirit, are all interconnected and is in tune with nature. They also believe that we can make use of the vibrational frequency coming from nature, alongside principles of natural law, as a means of healing our bodies and our emotions.

This concept can also be applied to the different physical aspects of the human body. For example, our kidney is linked to the sensory taste of salt, the tissue of our bones and teeth, the lower back, our ear, the knees, and our heels and feet. One affects the other —hence the need for holistic healing and holistic health. This interconnectedness isn't limited to just the physical, however.

Our emotional and mental state also affects different parts of our body.

For example, excess stress and suppressed emotions can affect our liver, and even cause imbalances. If you keep holding onto these emotions without expressing it, you might start feeling the effects in your liver. Stress can also affect heart health, directly impairing its proper function. This even has physical manifestations—I'm sure you're familiar with the tight feeling in your chest or the sudden rapid heartbeat that often accompanies stress and anxiety.

Aside from being a trigger to bad food habits, stress also affects our stomach health directly. It can cause imbalances, causing you to suffer from low metabolism and poor digestive health. Needless to say, if there's one big issue that we need to resolve, it would be stress. For many of us, however, our stressors tend to be things that are out of our control. For me, it was the numerous deadlines, the pressure from my environment, and my general lack of knowledge when it comes to properly managing all of that.

For you, it might be work and family commitments, your own personal expectations, different responsibilities, and frustrations that have piled up over the years. All of which are perfectly understandable—everyone, in some way, is burdened by something. But what we must realize is that there is a way of managing everything, to make sure that we are able to carry them well, and avoid unnecessary stresses that can lead to bad habits.

If we are to gain holistic health, we must nourish our bodies and our minds.

Below, I have compiled different stress management techniques that you can use. I made sure that the options I provide you with are not only accessible, but also viable even if you're a person who has plenty of responsibilities throughout the day. These take very little time, are affordable, and can be done even by beginners.

THE SECRETS OF TRADITIONAL CHINESE MEDICINE

With the help of traditional Chinese medicine, we can find effective and holistic ways of managing our stress levels. Instead of taking all sorts of medication meant to balance everything out, this ancient way of healing provides a great alternative to those looking for more natural methods of dealing with everyday stressors.

There are plenty of techniques, but I have compiled a short list for you. I made sure that these are accessible for everyone. Whether you're a family woman or man, a university student, or someone who has plenty of work-related stress, these are things that you can try to help improve your emotional and physical health.

Acupuncture.

This is one of the most common forms of treatment that has its roots in traditional Chinese medicine. It has proven benefits when it comes to healing the body and certain injuries, but did you know it can also treat stress?

Aside from causing us headaches, and digestion issues, stress also has a tendency to make our muscles tense. Leading to feelings of tightness in different parts of our bodies, particularly around the shoulder and the neck. No, it isn't just your sleeping position that could be causing this—it can also be due to pent up stress in the body that needs to be loosened up and released.

What acupuncture does is it opens up the meridian channels in our bodies, allowing energy or CHI to flow through properly. This, in turn, alleviates pain, and also improves the blood circulation throughout our bodies. With that, our muscles can relax better and we're no longer prone to aches and pains. With energy coursing through our bodies, we also feel lighter and clear-headed, and much less prone to giving into stress.

Healing Herbs.

When I first introduced the idea of traditional medicine, what was the first thing that came into your mind? It is likely that you pictured the use of natural remedies such as herbs. The Chinese certainly did not shy away from its use, creating concoctions that are meant to help balance the body and reduce stress. As we have emphasized earlier, Chinese Medicine thought of the physical, mental, and spiritual aspects of the self as a single organism. A good herbalist should be able to tell where your imbalances might be—thus it is important to consult with one if this is an option you're considering.

That said, let's talk about some of the herbs you should try.

Jujube seeds – These seeds are a well-known remedy that is used in traditional Chinese medicine for soothing the mind and reducing stress in the process. It can be taken in tea form and works best if you drink it before bed. These seeds are also used as an all-natural sleep aid.

Valerian root – This has been in use in Chinese medicine since ancient times and is most known for its ability to help people relax. In fact, even the Greeks used it for the same purpose. Much like jujube seeds, this can be taken as a tea before bed to help induce better sleep. The more rested you feel, the less prone you will be to stress.

Chrysanthemum tea – This is a staple, not just during mealtime, but for medicinal purposes as well. Chrysanthemum has been used in traditional Chinese medicine for thousands of years now and its main purpose is to help calm the mind, as well as keep the liver healthy. Two aspects of the body that are inherently connected and where balance must be maintained.

Green tea – This is known all over the world for its effective detoxifying and anti-inflammatory properties. However, it is also often used to help soothe the body and bring calmness to the mind. The best bit is that you can have it every meal and in lieu of your morning coffee. It will give you an energy boost in the process as well.

Kava root – Plenty of research has been done on this particular herb and all of them are consistent in stating that this is one of the most effective supplements for combating stress and anxiety. Not only can it tackle symptoms, it can even calm any anxious thoughts that you may have. It soothes muscle tension and spasms, restlessness, and can even aid with sleeplessness. It can be taken in capsule or table form, but you can also find it in liquid form.

Lemon balm – A daily dose of this, amounting to about 600mgs, is enough to help improve your mood, boost calmness, and help you maintain alertness. It is known to help people who are dealing with different mood disorders, aside from simply reducing stress. A cup of this every morning and every night should help you during more stressful days. So, instead of grabbing a soda or indulging in pizza, how about a nice pastry and some lemon balm to cap off your day?

You might be wondering, why bother with herbal teas when there are quicker remedies such as Valium, Xanax, and Ativan readily available? The answer is simple: these natural remedies come with no side-effects and no risk of you becoming overly dependent on them. As we have may clear early on, one of our goals is to also help you create better and healthier habits—so why add something that could be detrimental to your overall success and well-being? These teas work just as effectively, sometimes even better than big pharma medications. Give them a try and experience the benefits for yourself.

MEDITATION – THE REMEDY THAT COSTS $0

Let's quickly go over what meditation is. It is the practice of closing off the mind to environmental distractions, allowing us a type of internal and external pause. It also helps us detoxify the mind of any worries and stresses. For the purpose of holistic health and weight loss, you might think that there's no room for such a practice. After all, it involves staying still and simple breathing exercises. This is contrary to what most believe, that weight loss entails constant movement.

But as we have clarified previously, this is nothing more than a misconception.

Think of meditation like a steady stream of traffic. You're not moving along with it, but simply watching it flow pass. Now, imagine that traffic as a collection of all your stresses, your worries and anxieties, your fears— all the things that often trigger your bad food habits. Instead of responding to them and taking action like you normally would, just let them flow pass until they are out of sight.

GETTING STARTED WITH MEDITATION:

There are many different types of meditation, but for our purpose, what we require is something that will help manage stress and enable us to develop more mindfulness in our lives. Remember, meditation isn't about controlling or suppressing emotions—rather, it's acknowledging them in a way that's healthy for us. Here's how you can get started:

Breathing Meditation

This is something you can do during the mornings after you wake up and at night right before bed. You can make use of the habit link method to ensure that you'll be able to practice it on the daily. For example, in my case, I linked breathing meditation to my existing habit of stretching after my alarm goes off. After I do my morning stretches, I move to a quiet spot in my room (sometimes, I just stay on the bed) and practice meditation through breathing. It goes something like this:

Choose a quiet spot in your room, one that has very few distractions in it.

Set-up a cushion or anything that would make you feel more comfortable.

Next, count 1 to 5 between every inhale and exhale. This can take a bit of practice so don't rush yourself.

As you do this, your worries and stressors might begin to appear in your mind. Let this happen, but make sure that you do not linger on them. Acknowledge their presence, but focus on your breathing instead.

To close every meditation session, always give a word of thanks and do a bit of stretching before you prep for the day.

The first time you perform this breathing exercise, you can start with the most basic. Remember, if you're habit linking, always choose the easiest possible action which you can change later on. I suggest, simply sitting in bed while counting down 5 seconds between every inhale and exhale. Do this for 30 seconds for the first few days with the intention of increasing it later on.

How does this help? It adds a moment of pause to your day. Admit it, you are the type to rush through your mornings—going through every routine on auto-pilot and barely noticing that you've been acting on bad food habits. With the pause provided by meditation, you would be able to slowly plan out your day. During the breathing exercise, you are also able to deal with your emotions better. Instead of giving into the impulse and your cravings, you can pause and choose the better alternative.

Think of it as a pit stop of sorts, where you can pull yourself together and gather your bearings, before facing the day's challenges. The more prepared you are, the better you will be at handling different stressors.

YOUR GUIDE TO MINDFUL EATING

By now, you must have already heard about mindfulness—it is the current trend when it comes to wellness, after all. However, don't let its current trendiness deter you from giving it a shot. Fact is, this practice comes with plenty of benefits including: better sleep, boosting empathy, reducing your stress levels, and weight loss.

Yes, mindful eating is a very real thing.

Not only does it help you with stress management, it can also give you a much better relationship with food. Something that you need if you're looking to achieve holistic health and weight loss. By harnessing the power of mindfulness, you will also learn how to choose healthier foods and to treat food as a form of nourishment and not an emotional crutch. The latter is crucial to your heal and your weight goals.

How does it work?

Sometimes referred to as intuitive eating, this is simply the practice of being present whilst you eat. Basically, you have to give you full attention to observing what you're eating—the way it tastes, looks, smells, and even how it makes you feel. It's appreciating the process itself, without rushing through. Think of it in the same way as stopping to gaze at the sky or appreciate the way a mountain looks in the horizon—both things help heighten the experience of being in nature. Mindful eating works in the same way.

Look, I get it, we all often rush through our meals, whether that be in the morning or during lunch. For some, even dinner isn't a quiet time. The mere fact that we do this is actually bad for our health. Instead of being in the moment and appreciating the nourishing food before us, our mind wanders to all sorts of worries and anxieties. We are often distracted, mind racing from one thing to another. And as you all know, whenever our emotions are stressed, our digestive system suffers as well. Ever wonder why you sometimes feel bloated or lethargic after a meal? It isn't just the bad food, it's also your body telling you that your emotions are overwhelming it.

GETTING STARTED:

Always pause before you eat, then ask yourself why you're eating. One of the biggest components of mindful eating is actually understanding WHY you're eating. We have discussed that weight issues happen because people eat food, not because they need nourishment, but to help them deal with certain emotions that can be overwhelming.

What do you need to observe? Consider your environment, your current emotion or state of mind. You should also check yourself physically—do you feel hunger signals such as a rumbling stomach or lack of energy? Or do you simply want to procrastinate on work and distract yourself from the stress associated with your deadlines? It'll only take a few minutes but can spell the difference between eating for nourishment and eating out of habit.

Like mothers all over the world always say: Chew your food properly. Now, you might roll your eyes at this one, but hear me out. Eating too quickly, where you scarf down your food either out of habit or extreme hunger has many bad side effects. The biggest among them is the fact that it hinders proper digestion— the second, is the possibility of coming off as ill-mannered. Both things, you wouldn't want for yourself.

When you chew your food slowly and properly, not only do you get to savor it more, but you're also sending signals to your brain that makes it feel more satiated. In doing this, you can actually avoid overeating and avoid bloatedness after your meal.

Always eat without any distractions—and yes, that means turning off your TV or putting your phone away during meals. I get it, we've all become so used to eating whilst watching our favorite shows or whilst doing things on our phones. But did you know that this can lead to overeating, too?

Studies have shown that even the noise your food makes influences just how much you end up eating. Also referred to as the "Crunch Effect", it suggests that you're most likely to feel fuller sooner and eat less if you can hear the sound of yourself eating. So, remove your earphones and turn the TV off. Enjoy the quiet time you spend by yourself or with your family; this is a really beneficial habit to develop.

Now, this doesn't mean that you should be completely quiet

and stoic during mealtime. After all, such a thing is impossible especially if you have young kids around. Besides, for many families, mealtime is when they're able to discuss how their day went. The idea here is to keep your focus in the present and what better way to do that than being with family?

Always wait before you get second servings. Did you know that it takes your brain a total of 20 minutes before it receives the "message" that you're full? This is why it's so easy for people to overeat, especially if they have the habit of immediately getting up and going for another round of food.

Do your best to keep these in mind, whether you're eating at home or dining out with people. It can be very easy for you to overeat if you're dining out so this mindfulness becomes all the more important.

THE KEY TO STRESS JOURNALING

Every single day, we encounter a number of stressors—some are short term, whilst there are those that we have no real control over. For all of these, keeping a stress diary is not only helpful, but can also become a healthier outlet for releasing any pent up emotion we may have inside. As the name suggests, this is the practice of logging any stressful and anxious moments we encounter throughout the day.

The idea is that by keeping a record, we would be able to pinpoint the causes and provide solutions to each one so that we may be able to avoid experiencing the same stress again. It can also provide you with insight into your reactions to these stressors, allowing you to actually find the levels of pressure at which you're able to perform your best. Let's face it, not all stressors can be bad —some can push us into productivity, but there must always be a balance to it. A stress diary can help you figure that out.

How to Use It:

It is important that you make entries as regularly as possible throughout your day. It need not be every minute or even every hour, but you have to log any stressful incident that you experience. Here are the most important information you should include in your diary:

The date and time of the incident.

The stressful event you experience.

Your current mood or feeling. Include how happy you feel at the moment, using a scale of 0 to 10 with the 10 being the happiest you have been. You can be as succinct or as detailed when writing down your emotions.

How productive you are at the moment. Follow the same 0 to 10 scale, with 10 being the most productive you have been in a while.

Did the stressful feeling affected your appetite? Did you experience cravings and how did you react to it?

The fundamental cause of your stress. With this, be as objective and honest as you possibly can. This is also why writing immediately after the incident is key. If you leave it for later, chances are you'll lose the rawness of your emotion and any objectivity might become muddled by other distractions.

Other things you should include, but are not mandatory:

Symptoms you felt. This could include headaches, sweaty palms, increase pulse rate, and even butterflies in your stomach.

How well were you able to handle the situation? Did your reaction help solve the issue or did it only make it worse? Again, be as honest and objective as you can.

How to Analyze Your Diary:

Remember, you're not just journaling for the sake of getting your feelings out. It is also a way for you to properly analyze your stressors and your reaction to it, thus allowing you to improve. Here's a simple guide to help you study your notes:

First, take a closer look at all the stresses that you have experienced during the period you were writing in your diary. Make note of the most frequent stressors as well as the most unpleasant ones.

Next, study your personal assessments of the possible underlying causes for these stressors along with your appraisal of just how well you handled the associated situation. Are there obvious problems that need to be fixed? Are there things that can be improved? Make note of these as well.

Analyze the stressful situations in your diary and list all of the different ways these can be changed for the better.

Lastly, study how you felt during the times when you were under pressure. Study how it affected your productivity and your overall happiness. Try to explore if there is a middle ground for when you were under pressure, but still felt happy and were productive.

THE 4 A'S: AVOID, ALTER, ADAPT, ACCEPT

You, much like everyone else, know very well that there are certain stressors that happen in a very predictable pattern. This can occur during family gatherings, meetings, or during your commutes to work. The great thing about this predictable stressors is that you have the opportunity to change your reaction to it if you're unable to change the situation itself.

This is where the 4 A's come into play.

AVOID.

You must understand that avoiding a stressful situation that can be addressed properly is actually very unhealthy. Many people tend to do this; sweeping stressors under the rug and doing their best to ignore it until they can't anymore. However, many of the stressors in our everyday life can be resolved—we just need to be more observant and assertive towards them. Below are some examples:

It's alright to say NO. Whether in your personal or professional life, always know what your limits are and be firm enough to stick to them. For example, if you're working on developing better eating habits and you know that eating out with your friends causes you to overeat, it's alright to say NO to them.

You need not skip every single gathering or cut off all your friendships; it's about finding a balance. For example, do your friends or co-workers go out every night for some food and drinks? Perhaps you should try and limit yourself to joining them only a few days out of the week. Trust me when I say this: You will not be missing out anything by skipping a few night-outs and your friends will understand. In fact, you might even inspire them to develop healthier habits as well.

Take control of your environment. There are many things in our environment that can stress us out, but we need not put up with them all of time; certain things can be removed or replaced. For example, if you always end up buying bad food because you're distracted at the grocery, try doing it online instead. This way, you'll always have your list with you and you can choose online stores that only offer good food. If something on the television only adds to your feelings of anxiety, such as the news, turn it off and focus on something else.

Learn how to prioritize. Are you always feeling the pressure of being productive? You are not alone. Every single day, there are people who pile on task after task in order to keep themselves busy or make themselves appear to be so. The thing is, if you have too much on your plate, this will likely lead to STRESS. So, what can you do?

Let go of the need to be overly productive. Busy doesn't mean you're doing well—in fact, it could also be a sign of you trying to compensate for something else. Avoid taking on one too many things at a time and learn how to prioritize what needs to be worked on ASAP and what can be put off for later. This way, you have more free time and you feel less pressured as well.

ALTER.

It's a given fact that you won't always be able to avoid stressful situations. So, what can be done to the things you have zero control over? Do you just put up with them and hope you don't get sick from stress in the process? Of course not! What you can do is alter it—basically, change the way you operate and interact in your daily life.

Express your feelings, never bottle them up. Look, you're going to get nowhere if you keep mum about the things that are bothering you. There need not be a dramatic confrontation when it comes to expressing yourself; you can be assertive when communicating concerns, whether that be in your professional or personal life.

For example, if you've spent the weekday exhausted from work but your children are demanding that you take them somewhere fun during the weekend, it will save you a lot of stress to communicate your needs to them. Say that you need to rest and that you'll make it up to them another time. Keep in mind that unless you say something and explain, there will be people who won't understand your needs.

Should they still push you into going out, why not call a family member and see if they can bring the kids out with them instead? There are ways, don't let stress get to you.

Always be willing to compromise. If you're asking someone to change something for you, whether that be their behavior or schedule, you must also be willing to do the same. Through this, you and this person should be able to find neutral ground where you're both happy.

DO create a more balanced schedule. Now, this might seem a little tricky, but remember that all work and no play will lead to a major burnout—something that you want to avoid as much as possible because it can set you back in terms of productivity and when it comes to your health goals. So, what can you do? Make sure that you always have time for social activities, time for family, and some YOU-time. Everybody needs their piece of solitude every now and then. Pick up a hobby, something that will take your mind off of your stress and OFF of your cravings as well.

ADAPT.

In situations wherein you cannot alter the stressors you have, what can you do then? Well, you always have the option of adapting and regaining your sense of control by changing both your attitude and expectations. Now, before you say that this is impossible to do or that you'll only end up more stressed by trying it--- hear me out. Below is a short list of tips that you can try in order to make this happen.

Reframe your problems. When the stress hits, take a breath and shake your shoulders. Next, do your best to change your perspective of the situation and look at it from a more positive perspective. For example, instead of losing your wits whenever you encounter a traffic jam, take this time to meditate quietly. You can also listen to your favorite music, crack open a book, or simply zone out to help your mind find relaxation.

Try and see the bigger picture. Trust me when I say that there is always a bigger picture—begin by asking yourself how important the situation is in the long run. Will the thing that's stressing you out matter in a month or two? What about after a year? Thing is, once we consider the value of the stressor, we often discover that it amounts to very little. Sometimes, the thing stressing us out won't even matter after a day or two. So, is it really worth wasting your energy on getting upset? The simple answer is: NO. Focus your energy and your time elsewhere.

Practice gratitude. Too often, we forget to be thankful for what we have in life. No matter how small or difficult some of the challenges we face can be. We should also be thankful, not just for the material things, but also for the skills and positive qualities we have been gifted with. This may sound like such a simple strategy, almost too easy, but trust me when I say that it will help keep things in perspective. And as we have emphasized, perspective is KEY.

Adjust your standards. One of the major sources of stress in our lives is perfectionism. You may think that this only applies to your job, but that is certainly not the case. A lot of us aren't aware that we become perfectionists in our daily lives as well. From being unsatisfied with the way we look, the way our household is being run, the state of our finances, our relationships, and so on. We also look for perfection in the people around us, our family and our friends. By demanding perfection in the different aspects of our lives, we also set ourselves up for failure. So, what do we do? Set more reasonable standards for yourself and for others. Learn and understand that "good enough" is okay.

ACCEPT.

There is no denying the fact that life can throw us major curveballs at times—the same applies to stressors. There will be those that cannot be avoided at all. Such is the case when someone we love passes away or if our finances take a hit due to economic factors that is out of our control. Accepting these things will be difficult, but compared to the other options? It certainly is the best for us in the long run. Instead of trying to go against it or burning ourselves out with overthinking, we must learn how to let go and accept—then move on.

Learn forgiveness. It's so easy for people to harbor negative and toxic feelings whenever something wrong is done on them or whenever things don't go their way. In accepting that we live in an imperfect world and we are all imperfect in many ways, we also learn to forgive these things and manage to let go of any resentments. For example, you must forgive yourself for any shortcomings you feel you might have. Perhaps you weren't able to exercise as regularly as you wanted or indulged your cravings after a stressful week. Forgive yourself for these things then move on so you may start anew. Lingering on the bad only heightens your stress further and isn't going to be healthy for you in any way.

Don't try to control what is uncontrollable. Are you the type to be very controlling of everything that goes on around you? Well, here's a bit of bad news: Your efforts, though valiant in some way, is futile. See, there are many things that we won't be able to control and among those are the behavior of other people. This includes, not just your co-workers, but also your family. The people you're in a relationship with. Your friends. Sure, you might not love them less, but you are adding unnecessary stress to your life and theirs by trying to control things. Instead of hyper-focusing on what's beyond your control, focus your energy on what can be changed and make it better—such as your reaction to stressful situations.

Always look for the upside. Everyone faces seeming insurmountable challenges in their life; whether that be in work, in love, family, or even health—the difference lies in how we handle them. Do you try your best to see the challenges as necessary for growth or do you only see them as personal failures? If they are due to your own choices, you must learn forgiveness then reflect on your actions. Even in our worst days, there are still lessons to be learned.

WORKSHEET:

AVOID	ALTER	ADAPT	ACCEPT

Using the template above, categorize your stressors according to your ability to deal with them. Are they avoidable? Can you alter them in anyway? And so on. The idea here is to put things into perspective; in labeling each one, you'll also be able to see that things aren't as bad as you think they are. That there is still something you can do, even if that "something" calls for no real action on your part.

Don't do this as a one-time thing, however. Start by writing things down once a week or more if you find it's needed. It will really give you better insight into your own situation.

WEEK 4:

THE BITTER TRUTH ABOUT SUGAR—

Previously, we have discussed the concept of building better habits and the different stress management techniques we can use to help bring balance to our lives. By now, you should have been able to put what you have learned into practice and seen some of the benefits it can bring into your life. This time, we'll be tackling nutrition—another important aspect of holistic weight loss.

In talking about this topic, we cannot overlook the role that the food and health industry play in it. That said, I present you with the 3 most common misconceptions that people have about it.

FOOD AND HEALTH INDUSTRY: DEBUNKED

Healthcare wants you to be healthy.

Let me begin by giving you the hard facts: Healthcare in the United States is largely privatized. What I'm trying to say is that it's all one big business that's profiting from people being sick. Sure, you might think this is crazy, but look at it a little more closely:

With your weight gain came other complications such as diabetes, so you go to your doctor for medication that would help with it. Now, your doctor will likely write up a prescription for you which you'll need to get filled at the pharmacy. I'm sure you've been appalled by the cost of medicine before--- you're not alone. Still, much like everyone else, you go ahead and buy it because it's meant to HEAL YOU. It's meant to HELP YOU.

But pull away the curtain and you'll find that behind the cure, there's a huge industry that's designed to make money for hospital providers, insurance companies, and the big pharmaceuticals who provide the meds. What I'm trying to say is that they're all trying to make money—by taking way too much from you. They are profiting while people keep on getting sick. The cure they offer? Temporary.

Americans spend twice the amount of money on health care when compared to other developed countries, but also end up last in rank when it comes to the quality of services provided.

Here are some key US Healthcare facts to help put that in perspective:

Back in 1969, the American Healthcare industry was worth $24.7 billion. Currently, in 2019, it is now worth $3.504 TRILLION. Imagine the huge leap it made within a few decades. All of that, coming from the average person's wallet—the same people suffering, not just from their illness but from struggling with having to spend so much for a cure. It shouldn't be that way. You know it. Everyone knows it.

If you ever have a heart attack and need to receive hospital care, be prepared to pay $20,246 in costs. The amount alone would be enough to give any person yet another heart attack--- especially so if they are living from wage to wage, which is what the average person on the US does. They are the most vulnerable among us.

It's no wonder than 1.4 million Americans actually went overseas to seek medical care, knowing that even if they spend money on airfare, they will still get a better deal.

Speaking of which, did you know that the anti-cancer drug Avastin is ten times more expensive in the US than it is in the UK?

Going back to the topic of weight, about 4 out of 10 Americans are morbidly obese. On top of that, 7 out of 10 are overweight. As you can imagine, this can lead to a whole other list of complications and illnesses that requires medication—even more money funneling into the Healthcare business.

Last, but not the least, about 9.1% of Americans were not covered by health insurance according to 2017 statistics. The most common reason for which is that they found healthcare to be unaffordable, whilst others felt that they did not need it.

Did you know that pharmacies can charge people whatever prices they want for the meds, no matter how ridiculously expensive that number is, because of lobbyists? If you study it closer, there really is no logic no proper reasoning when it comes to how they charge for prescriptions. In the past, pharmaceutical companies attributed the steep prices of their medications to innovation— the argument is that continuously improving and creating new drugs also means higher costs. However, new studies reveal that this isn't the case at all.

The study suggests that the costs have gone up because the big pharms are actually raising the price of drugs that are already available. That doesn't make sense, right? If it's new innovations that's raising the cost, then why are the costs for old medicines still going up? Again, a lack of logic. Between 2008 and 2016 alone, many brand name oral prescription drugs increased in price at about 9% annually. The injectables increased by 15% every year. Inflation, on the other hand, increased by only 2%.

Something simply doesn't add up.

Just take Lantus for example. This is a Sanofi band insulin that has increased in price by almost 50% even though it has been in the market for more than 10 years. And with so many obese and overweight people suffering from diabetes needing this insulin, the struggle and difficulty they face when it comes to obtaining them increases as well.

Still unconvinced? Let me tell you my story.

I went for a routine annual checkup last year and I thought myself smarter for having experienced getting overcharged in the past. This time, I was very cautious about the process and made sure that I spoke to my insurance and my doctor beforehand to make it clear that insurance was covered for my visit. What this means is that I need not pay for anything out of my own pocket.

On the day of my check-up, I even made sure that I was only there for a regular visit—this was how wary I was of getting extra charges billed to me. The doctor confirmed and we began. All was well until she pointed out that I had a minor rash on my stomach. Of course, out of curiosity. I asked a few questions about what it might mean. The doctor confirmed that it was nothing serious, but she did offer me a prescription which I declined politely.

Fast forward to a few weeks later, when I go to check my mail and find a letter from my insurance provider. Now, you can guess just as well as I did that I had been charged extra during my visit. There was an extra $75 on my bill, which I phoned my insurance carrier for to ask how that could have happened. They explained that I was charged for a separate procedure just because I asked a couple of questions about the skin rash.

Needless to say, this proves that healthcare is completely driven by greed and profit—if my story, one that resonates with other people's experiences, does not drive the point home then I don't know what will.

So, what is the point of this all? Well, think back to the previous module where we talked about how weight gain isn't just cosmetic, but is also associated to common chronic health issues such as diabetes, inflammation in the joints, and a slew of other disorders. What I'm trying to do is help you save money and keep you from having to go through the same healthcare issues that I did. The facts don't lie: getting sick in the United States can leave you bankrupt—it can put you under such heavy debt that you'll be working to pay for the rest of your life.

Ask yourself, do you want to live that way? I'm sure the answer is NO.

The recommended food guidelines are up to date.

It's so easy for us to trust the food guidelines provided by authorities on the subject, believing that they know what's best for us and have our best interest in mind. However, this is not always the case and many of the recommended food guidelines we have is actually outdated. The most notable example would be the USDA Food Pyramid, a well-known diagram that you'll surely recognize as it's been ingrained in our head whilst we were growing up.

Here's a refresher, if you need one. The diagram itself is quite easy to understand. You'll find your whole wheat and grains at the very bottom. This means that they are the staples you should eat a lot of. Next, you have your fruits and veggies—food items that you also need a good amount of in your diet. Moving further up, you'll find seafood and different meats. At the very top, within the smallest triangle, are the fats and oils which you should consume very little of.

So, what do I mean when I say it's outdated? I refer to the idea that we all fat is bad. This is a movement that started back in the 1960's, where the "low fat" phenomena really took hold in everyone's consciousness.

I have very vivid memories of this as a child. Back when my mother would cook chicken drumsticks or thighs, and each time I would try to eat the skins she would stop me from doing so because it wasn't healthy. Because the skin contained a lot of fat. Of course, this made me a little sad as the skin had the most flavor. Even until recently, I did my best to avoid having butter because of the notion that "fat is bad". Growing up, I believed that fat would cause someone to become overweight.

This belief created a calorie gap which needed to be filled and that is where grains enter the picture. With grains, there was a surge in our carb intake which helped satisfy our daily caloric needs. The carbs we introduced in our daily diet came in the form of grains and wheat. Now, looking at the current stats, you'll see that there was still an increase in cases of fatty liver, obesity, and even arthritis issues despite the shift in everyone's diet.

This was furthered by the argument that whole grain is better than white bread. What we did not see is that the food industry was profiting significantly by changing the way we consumed food. They saw the huge opportunity to make more money by developing cheaper processed foods that used a lot of flour, wheat, high fructose syrup, and corn starch. As long as it was labeled as "low fat" people bought it, thinking that it was better for their health. Just take Kraft for example. The company had a whopping 1800% increase in their total revenue since the 80s. And do you really think the food they offer is good for you?

It doesn't end there, however. Did you know that some of the most respected non-profit food organizations, such as the American Diabetic Association, who talk about how certain foods are healthier than others, are actually funded by Big Pharmaceuticals and Big Food companies? How can you trust their opinion then? ADA itself is supported by Novo Nordisk and Eli Lily, two big pharm companies. These two companies have pledged over 11 million in 2014 alone.

The same applies to medical centers that have cushy relationships with the medical device industry and big pharms. You cannot completely trust the data being published, because they could very easily be withholding important information—as transparent as these studies might seem, many of them are only cleverly disguised marketing campaigns. Take for example the studies done on antidepressants. Those with positive results have 37 out of 38 different trials published. Not a bad number, right? Well, consider this: if the results are negative, 33 out of 36 trials are NOT published.

So, what's the takeaway from all of this?

Be more cautious about what you believe in. If you read a new study being conducted on how food X is better than food Y, always take it with a grain of salt. Look into who did the study, who wrote the article, and so on. Doing your own research will help make sure that you get to the bottom of things and if you ever decide to give the diet a try, you have full confidence in what you're doing. If you find a food study is being funded by a big pharm company—better think twice about buying into it.

To Recap:

In this module, you have learned about the two biggest misconceptions when it comes to the healthcare and food industry. Here's a quick refresher before we move on:

It is a misconception that the healthcare industry is a helping hand that will pull you out of your health struggles. Keep in mind that the method they use for "helping" you merely treats the symptoms and not the actual root of the disease. Note that they also get money whenever an expensive procedure is one on you — so the more procedures done and the more expensive it is, the more profitable it is for them.

Instead of asking you what may have caused your illness, they go straight to prescribing you with medication, which leads to more profits for them. Here's a fact: Healthcare is a business, the biggest one in the US, which profits through people's illnesses.

The food industry is no different and many of what you used to believe about food is outdated or a propaganda by the people running things behind the scenes. Many of the food studies being done today, in order to find the healthiest for us, is also funded by major players in the food industry as well as the big pharms. Needless to say, you cannot completely trust any of the published results.

It is my hope that you have a better perspective on both healthcare and the food industry after this module. This is so that you'll also be more assertive when it comes to the information you'll be putting your trust in and be more aware of the influence big pharmaceuticals have on these different industries.

As a consumer, you need to take charge of your own health. You've already taken the first steps by learning more and exploring all the options you have. What comes next is to start healing your body and that begins with the food you consume.

OUR PRIMITIVE ANCESTORS AND THEIR DIET

This time, you'll learn about the two distinct shifts in human history that subsequently led to a shift in our way of eating, as well as an increase in various diseases.

To start, let's take a step back to 100,000 years before modern times. This will bring you to a time where forests are lush and abundant, where you can observe a primitive tribe going through their daily activities. The males would go out to hunt at the crack of dawn, taking weapons with them. The females, on the other hand, would go in search of fruits and berries, all whilst looking after the children. This was a time when access to sugar was limited and everything they needed to eat were either hunted or foraged by hand. This is common among all the primitive tribes of the world. Whenever they hunted an animal, they wasted very little of it. They didn't just go for the lean meat like modern man would. Instead, they are all the organs and fats.

Think of it this way: after having risked their lives and exerted a lot of energy into catching the animal, do you think they would just go for the leanest part of it and throw the rest away? Despite that, there were no autoimmune diseases, heart diseases, and obesity issues. These illnesses were unknown to societies that followed traditional diets and I'm talking about globally. Just look at the Maori of New Zealand, the native North Americans, and the Kitavan of Papua New Guinea—you will see that none of their people had these issues.

BMIs of 20 were normal—in this case, think of BMI as a rough proxy for obesity. Anything that's around 25 is considered to be borderline overweight. These people, despite not having access to the dental care we do today, also had healthy teeth. Their blood pressures were normal and they did not experience acid reflux or bloating.

DOMESTICATION

Now comes the first major shift. This happened about 300 generations ago when our ancestors discovered that it was possible to domesticate certain animals. Think of this as our ancestors taming wild animals in order to keep them in a "farm". For example, we began domesticating the cows and pigs because they were not dangerous. As time went on and because of domestication, the cows became smaller and smaller. We began to live closer to them as well hence also developed their diseases.

Our ancestors also observed the eating patterns of these domesticated animals. If they are grass then perhaps we could do it as well? They tried, through much trial and error, then learned the hard way that it isn't possible. Of course, each trial came with bouts of abdominal pain, nausea, and other issues. That is how we learned to avoid them.

AGRICULTURE

It is through that trial and error that our ancestors discovered that we can eat the seeds of grasses. This is where the second major shift happens. By separating them from the husk, drying, and then crushing the seeds with hard stones they could be made edible. If heated with water—they ended up with the first porridge.

Fast forward to some thousands of years later, the Egyptians learned how to make beer through the fermentation process. In learning how to make beer, they also developed a method of making leavened bread. This is a very critical period for humans as this is when we began to rely on grains—basically, the seeds of grasses.

These two shifts, domestication and agriculture, really were the biggest departures from man's primitive diet. They only happened about 10,000 years ago, accounting for only about 1% of our human history. Within that span of time, however, there was a significant increase in the development of various health issues. This includes iron deficiency, crooked teeth, a reduction in bone length (leading to shorter heights), just to name a few.

Remember how our primitive ancestors avoided grasses because it made them sick YET the generations that came after began eating its seeds anyway? It's no wonder that the incidence of diseases increased during that time. Our ancestors knew better by staying away from the grasses and relying on foraged food instead.

GOOD GRAIN, BAD GRAIN – WHICH IS WHICH?

Now, I know you might be wondering why our more recent ancestors (think 1 to 2 generations ago) seemed to be healthier than most of us. Looking at pictures of humans from about 100 years ago show that they were thinner despite consuming grains. One of the main reasons that should be pointed out is that the grains they had then and even back during the medieval times, were different from what we eat today. I'll tell you more about this in the next lessons—for now, meditate on the fact that it is only over the last fifty years where food hybridization became common place.

TO RECAP:

Alright, here's another refresher. In this lesson, you have learned that our eating habits have changed significantly over the generations. There were two big shifts: domestication and agriculture.

Between these two, it is agriculture that really changed the game for us—humans began to rely more on grain consumption for their dietary needs. Because of this and because of the demand that needed to be met, we began to genetically modify wheat. This helped us produce more of it and it made the plant more resistant to diseases. In doing that, however, we opened a pandora's box of chronic diseases that modern man is struggling to combat. The biggest of it all? Obesity.

SUGAR IS NOT NATURAL

When it comes to the things you must cut out from your diet, sugar certainly tops the list.

The average American consumes about 200 pounds of sugar per year. Many of them believe that sugar is, in fact, natural. However, this isn't the case. Remember, natural does not equal, naturally-occurring. In nature, sugars are locked up in the fibrous externals of a vegetable.

With that in mind, let's talk about naturally-occurring sugar vs. added sugar.

What are added sugars? These are sugars that are added to food during processing and includes the likes of: high-fructose corn syrup, white sugar, and slightly healthier options (often described as natural, but certainly not naturally-occurring) such as honey, maple syrup, and coconut sugar. These "natural" options are better than table sugar, but note that they still need to be consumed in small amounts.

Then you have naturally-occurring sugar from fruit such as apples and berries, or ones found in some veggies such as sweet potatoes and beets. These are seen as better and healthier options if you want something sweet—but what makes it different?

It's in how it impacts our body. For example, a spoonful of table sugar, when added to your food causes inflammation and then quickly turns to fat if you don't use it up as fuel. On the other hand, you have something like a cup of berries which contains 15 grams of naturally-occurring sugar alongside other important nutrients that actually influences the way our body breaks down its sugar content.

For example, fiber found in fruits helps with slowing down digestion to prevent a blood-sugar spike. Yogurt has proteins that enables the body to process these natural sugars at a much slower pace. And that's not even counting all the other good stuff you get from eating fruits, which includes: probiotics, minerals, and a number of vitamins that will benefit your health. You get none of that from table sugar or even those added to sweeten various processed food products.

Do we really need sugar in our diet, outside of the naturally-occurring ones? Truth be told, we do not need added sugar in our daily diets. Remember that our primitive ancestors were able to live well enough even without root crops and fruits—they got all of their energy from fats. It's actually protein that we really need, not fat, but the latter provides us with a viable solution should proteins become scarce. That said, we have no real need for carbohydrates as well.

Think about it. If we really needed carbohydrates in our daily diet, then people who have been doing Ketogenic diets, Atkins, Paleo, and every other low carb diet would likely suffer and become sick. But they don't—in fact, they get even healthier. Now, this doesn't mean that you shouldn't eat any sugar at all. Rather, what you should do is limit your intake of it to natural sources such as foods. The most important thing to remember is that even in healthy foods such as fruits, you must also practice moderation. These are not meant to be eaten in unlimited quantities—certain fruits can have too much sugar and can still be bad for you if you don't practice moderation.

The best fruits to eat are berries because they have high antioxidant content. You should avoid items such as dried fruits as these have high sugar content. Lastly, do be careful when eating honey as well. Make sure you only do so in moderation.

SUGAR IS KILLING YOU – HERE'S HOW:

We've established the fact that sugar is not something that was common food for our primitive ancestors. In fact, it is mostly unnatural and impacts our body negatively. Here are some of the ways it does that:

Increases blood sugar.

When that sweet, sugary donut first enters your body, your bloodstream experiences a spike in sugar levels because of it. As a result of this, your pancreas begin to secrete a hormone called insulin. Its job is to regulate the amount of sugar in your bloodstream, it directs the cells to absorb the sugar as energy, thus lowering its levels in your blood. This sounds harmless until you develop insulin resistance.

What is insulin resistance? Well, imagine this: you habitually indulge your cravings for sweets whenever stress happens. This means that your blood sugar is constantly increasing and your pancreas are consistently producing insulin to help balance things out. After some time, your cells will fail to respond to the insulin—basically, insulin resistance. A little confusing? Here's a helpful analogy to aid you in understanding.

Have you ever had a friend who constantly asks for your help? Maybe it's for something as simple as advice, perhaps it's something more annoying such as borrowing money or asking to be driven somewhere. The first few times were okay, but then they begin to ask you more and more. After a while, you begin to ignore them. They were simply asking for way too much and you are tired of it. Insulin resistance is a bit like this—the cells ignore the direction from the insulin because it happens way too often.

What comes next is the nothing short of terrible—you see, with the cells not taking in the sugar in your blood you end up with very high blood sugar levels. This, by itself, is problematic enough but it also leads to something worse. Because your cells are not using the sugar for energy, they turn to the fat and protein reserves in your body. To get to those, however, they have to go through your bloodstream. Think of it this way: the fat and protein stores in your body are now traversing the bloodstream highway to get to your cells. This means that there's a LOT more bad fats, such as LDL, collecting in your bloodstream that can lead to serious illnesses.

With that in mind, you might want to rethink having a second donut the next time you get a craving.

Tooth Decay

As you already know, everything in our body is interconnected. That also applies to the increase of blood sugar levels. First off, it causes fluctuations which affects the calcium and phosphorus ratios in our blood. This leads to our body needing to pull more calcium from our teeth and bones as a means of compensating. So, the more blood sugar fluctuations you have and the more inconsistent they are, the likelier your chance is at developing tooth decay since you're losing calcium from your tooth.

So if you thought that its carbs or food bacteria that's causing your teeth to decay, you're wrong. It's this imbalance in your blood ration chemistry that's really damaging your pearly whites. Later, we'll discuss more about fructose which has far worse effects— it can lead to fatty liver, inflammation, and an increase in blood triglycerides. Basically, all of the bad stuff. In fact, research shows that fructose is ten times more potent than glucose as a glycation agent—so much for those healthy treats such as dried dates, raisins, and fruit smoothies.

SUGAR AND DAMPNESS ACCORDING TO TCM

TCM or Traditional Chinese Medicine recognizes different factors and influences that affect both physical and energetic systems of our bodies. This includes wind, heat, and dampness.

Dampness is a condition that exists within our bodies; it is a reflection of dampness as it occurs naturally. It arises in our bodies through several ways. The first of which could be because of our digestive system's inability to transport fluids. It can also be because our body is overwhelmed by external damp, one that comes directly from our environment such as damp weather and damp-producing foods.

Dampness can also arise as a response to being sick and from overusing different medication such as antibiotics. These are known to promote dampness. How does dampness manifest in our bodies? Well, the most recognizable form of it would be Phlegm. Here's what you need to keep in mind when it comes to dampness appearing in our bodies:

When dampness is caused by issues with our digestion, it often ends up in the lungs and in our large intestine. When dampness moves into our lungs, the most common symptom is the presence of phlegm while coughing—something that happens whenever we eat things that are difficult to digest such as greasy food or cold dairy products.

When dampness moves to the large intestine, we experience different intestinal disturbances which manifests as loose stools or diarrhea. Even intestinal rumblings can be attributed to dampness in our bodies. TCM considers dampness as a contributing factor to many illnesses, including: high cholesterol, metabolic disorders, cancer, chronic fatigue syndrome, eczema, MS, allergies, fibromyalgia, and environmental illness.

EXTERNAL VS. INTERNAL DAMPNESS

The most common of the two would be internal dampness and

can combine with either heat or cold to produce damp-heat or damp cold. Its symptoms include puffiness of the skin, an overall feeling of heaviness, water retention or swelling, phlegm discharge, distended abdomen, loose bowels, nodular masses, and so on. People who are experiencing this condition tend to be low in energy and also gain weight easily.

On the other hand, you have external dampness which is basically a prolonged condition of high humidity and typically occurs during the late summer season or in early autumn. It may also be prevalent during long-lasting rainy weather. The most common symptoms reported by people who have experienced it include, joint soreness and pain, as well as a heavy sensation in both head and body. There are those who also reported dizziness and discharges that form on the body, such as thrush, suppurating sores, and weeping eczema.

THE ROLE OF SUGAR IN DAMPNESS

Poor diet plays a significant role when it comes to a person developing internal dampness. Constantly consuming foods that impair digestion, interfere with spleen processes, and yield food stagnation all contribute to internal dampness. Some of the most common foods that causes this include: milk products with the exception of yogurt, white-wheat flour, sugar and sweets, an excess of raw fruits, an excess of mushrooms and fungi, processed starch products, cold beverages, peppers, and raw vegetables. An excess of fermented foods, especially those containing vinegar and yeast also contribute to this.

Since poor diet is one of the main causes for dampness, switching to a better one will certainly help with treatment. It is also important to understand the importance of the spleen since it affects our body's ability to heal as well as its overall immunity. Cutting sugar from your diet is a step in the right direction and you're likely to feel its positive effects immediately. Sugar is one of the major disruptors when it comes to the spleen functions, but it is also the most common craving people have whenever stressed.

That said, the sweetness it provides isn't completely bad for the spleen. In fact, in small amounts, it can be beneficial. This means a sweet potato that's been mashed with just a pinch of brown sugar and some butter—that's enough to keep your spleen happy and operating properly. See, the key here is balance. Finishing an entire bag of peanut butter cups? Definitely not balance. In fact, it would likely leave you feeling completely fuzzy and swampy.

There are also damp clearing foods and fruits that you can try to help get rid of that swampy feeling. Add more onion, radish, daikon radish, lettuce, corn, turnip, scallion, alfalfa, umeboshi plum, and unsweetened cranberry to your diet. Having more beans such as mung beans and aduki beans are known to be very potent when it comes to clearing damp. The best bit is that you can produce so many different dishes from just these two so it wouldn't be hard to incorporate them into your daily diet.

SUGAR MAKES YOU AGE FASTER

Aside from being a major factor when it comes to the development of chronic illnesses, did you know that sugar can also make you age much faster?

Glycation

To add to the neverending list of bad things that happen to the body because of too much sugar, we have what's called Glycation. This is a chemical reaction between the proteins and sugars in your body. Think of it this way:

Imagine a hamburger patty. Now, before you cook it, the patty is soft and pink. It turns brown and firmer once you set it on the grill—basically losing its softness. This is similar to what happens inside your body during glycation. The sugars attack your proteins, acting like leeches that latch onto the proteins and slowly break them down. This makes them stiffer and much less flexible—your muscles get harder and also a lot more fragile.

Even scarier is the fact that glycation can occur anywhere in our body that has protein. It can happen in the protein lenses in our eyes where cataracts and floaters eventually develop. It can also happen in our skin where glycation creates wrinkles and age spots all over. We can also experience arthritis and joint pain if it happens in our cartilage proteins. Then you have glycation in the kidneys which can lead to organ failure. Glycation in the brain can lead to demention and glycation in the LDL particles in our bloodstream can cause heart disease.

Like I've said, its effects is nothing short of devastating.

ADVANCED GLYCATION PRODUCTS

Glycation creates what's known as AGE's or Advanced Glycation products in our bodies. These eventually accumulate in the body's proteins which renders them deformed and brittle. But they don't just occur in our bodies, we can also end up consuming them unknowingly as well. They are found in foods that have been deep fried, especially ones that have been browned. I know, you're thinking about that golden-brown chicken skin but hear me out first.

It's already been established that you must avoid fried foods as much as possible. You should also avoid barbecuing your meat too much and eliminate processed foods from your life. Needless to say, what you need to do in order to reduce your intake of AGEs is to choose better and healthier cooking methods. Again, finding balance is key. If you cannot remove fried foods from your diet, make sure you cut down on it as much as possible instead.

Fructose

If you thought the above was the worst of it, you thought wrong. There is another type of glycation involving fructose that is much worse. Fructose as you may or may not know is another type of sugar—but the worst possible kind. Think of it as the Darth Vader of sugars. It is also commonly found in plenty of processed and packaged foods. In fact, grab something from your fridge, like a soft drink and you're likely to find "high fructose corn syrup" on the ingredients list. While you're at it, pour that drink down the drain.

Aside from increasing insulin production and making blood sugars surge significantly, fructose actually delays the effect by several days. Like a Trojan horse, it very sneakily increases your blood sugar levels and also increases triglyceride particles in your bloodstream—often leading to heart disease. It also contributes to increasing blood pressure, visceral fat, inflammation, and even fatty liver.

Fructation is the worst kind of glycation as it is faster and can lead to a slew of serious illnesses such as cancer, dementia, and heart disease.

So, what should you do? Well, the first step is to limit your consumption of fructose to only those found in fruits. Later, we'll cover the just how much fruit you should consume as well as some of the most common misconceptions about it. Needless to say, there is plenty. Remember, just because something is natural or organic, it doesn't immediately mean that it would be good for you. Just take fruits as one example.

Trust me on this for I once made the mistake of believing that it's okay to consume fruits in large amounts because they're supposed to be good for me. Because of that mistake, I managed to contract a severe case of bronchitis in the process. I dealt with a hacking cough that was so persistent, I even had trouble sleeping. From there, I made yet another mistake—I took honey and lemon to soothe my throat. Whilst these are very healthy when consumed moderately, I had so much of it that it affected my health further. By the end of it all, I developed a little extra floater because of glycation.

BEVERAGES

So, did you really pour that soda down the drain or did you end up drinking it? Did you know that sugary beverages are the most common culprits for the abovementioned issues? Sugar-sweetened beverages, also known as SSBs, are the top sources for added sugars when it comes to the American diet. SSBs are basically any liquid that is sweetened with various types of sugars, including: sucrose, molasses, raw sugar, maltose, lactose, malt syrup, high-fructose corn syrup, glucose, honey, corn sweetener, dextrose, corn syrup, and brown sugar.

Ssbs are also not limited to just regular soda. There are also fruit drinks, energy drinks, sports drinks, coffee, sweetened waters, and tea beverages that have added sugar in them. Needless to say, it pays to check the ingredients of what you're buying. Frequently drinking these are directly linked to kidney disease, type 2 diabetes, weight gain and obesity, non-alcoholic liver disease, gout, tooth decay, and heart disease. Despite knowing all these things, however, portion sizes for sugary drinks have increased significantly over the past 40 years and this has lead to an increase in consumption among children and adults as well.

Here are some interesting facts to note:

Prior to the 1950s, the standard bottles were no bigger than 6.5 ounces. Come the 1950s, however, soda companies introduced larger sizes, including the 12-ounce can we are familiar with today. This became available to most of the population by the 1960s. 20-ounce plastic bottles were the norm by the 1990s and today, you can even get soft-drinks in 1-liter bottles.

In 1999 to 2004, the average children and youth in the US can average up to 224 calories per day from sugary beverages alone, taking up nearly 11% of their daily intake. This number only saw an increase the following, even beating our pizza when it came to the top calorie source in most teen's diet. In fact, from 1989 to 2008, calorie intake from sugary beverages increased by over 60% among preteens.

It isn't just in the US, however. All over the world, especially in developing countries, the consumption of sugary drinks is on the rise due to urbanization and beverage marketing.

5 out of 10 adults drink a sugar sweetened beverage each day. Among adults, SSB consumption is higher among males.

Drinking a single 12-ounce can of soda per day can effectively increase your risk of dying from heart disease by almost one-third. Those who drink 1 to 2 sugary beverages per day also have a 26% higher risk of developing type 2 diabetes when compared to those who drink less than 1 every month.

What makes liquid sugar more dangerous than, say, your regular table one? Well, the big difference is how easy it can be to overconsume sugary beverages. To put that in perspective, you can easily consume 9 teaspoons of sugar by drinking one soda —that's twice as many sugars in an apple. The worst part is that people barely even notice what they're doing. Now, imagine drinking two cans a day. Maybe even three. After all, aren't these drinks marketed as the best companions for every meal?

And that's another thing. Beverage companies spend billions in order to market these drinks, targeting the most vulnerable age groups, which are between 2 to 17 years old. It should be no surprise then that the statistics reflect this—the biggest soda drinkers are children and the youth. Now, big soda companies such as Coca-Cola do acknowledge their role when it comes to the obesity issues within this age group and in 2013, they launched an anti-obesity advertisement. They promoted calorie-free beverages and encouraged people to take responsibility when it comes to their drink choices and weight.

The responses to this were mixed, with many experts pointing out how inaccurate and misleading the campaign was when it came to stating the real dangers of soda. This takes us back to big companies funding food related studies and how that can taint the results being published to the public. In this case, the studies funded by the beverage industry was found to be about eight times more likely to publish results that favor the industry itself. Propaganda at its finest.

SUGAR FREE IS JUST AS BAD

Just because something is being marketed as being the "better option" it doesn't mean that it is. Anyone can plaster a "healthier" label on any food item and people who don't do their research will snap it up. This has proven to be true for "sugar free" or "low calorie" drinks. What most people don't realize is that whilst it does contain few to no calories at all, it also has a higher concentration of sweetness per gram when compared to the regular sweetened drinks.

This is because their use artificial sweeteners such as sucralose and aspartame, as well as plant extracts such as monk fruit, glycosides, and steviol. If you didn't know yet, aspartame along with other non-nutritive sweeteners can directly affect your body weight as it actually increases your appetite. So when you drink these "sugar free" drinks whilst having your meals, you are more likely to eat more than what's necessary. Consumed in large doses (900 to 3,000mg a day) it can also cause headaches especially in people who are already susceptible to migraines.

So, what's the best alternative?

WATER IS STILL THE BEST OPTION

It may taste like nothing, but it is the best for your health. However, there is something you should know when it comes to drinking water—it is best served warm. The Chinese have been drinking their water this way for thousands of years, even today where cold and refreshing water is readily accessible. Regardless of the weather, they drink warm water instead of something that's been chilled.

So, what's the science behind it?

A healthy child or adult has an internal core body temperature of about 37 degrees Celsius. If this increases by just 2 degrees, the body would begin showing signs of fever. With that in mind, TCM suggests that we are creating an opposite effect by regularly drinking iced fluids. However, the body will not show signs similar to that of a fever. Instead, the effect is spread over many years, initially affecting our metabolism and digestion before it begins to show negative effects in our organs. In TCM, "cold" points to any drink that is less than 37 degrees Celsius. It is suggested that we drink warm to hot water—just make sure it's not too hot that it will burn your tongue or make you sweat.

There are many benefits to doing this as everyday practice. Here are a few to note:

It helps with protecting and preserving our internal organs. It can also promote a smoother blood circulation. Did you know that drinking refrigerated water is no different from putting your organs in a freezer? This results in contractions and slows down the processes of your organs so that they're not functioning at their fullest.

Cold water also blocks our body's meridian channels and congeals blood circulation. Brain freeze is just one example of this principle.

It can remedy disharmonious internal cold patterns. In order to maintain holistic health, we must also maintain balance in our internal body temperature. However, drinking cold liquids can disrupt that. When this happens, we experience internal cold syndrome and its symptoms include: cold hands and feet, painful periods for women, Raynaud's phenomenon, weak appetite, varicose veins, abdominal pain, poor digestion, weight gain, loose stools, depression, chronic fatigue, chronic pain, and arthritic pain.

Eating spicy foods can remedy this, but the most efficient treatment would be switching to hot water.

Helps with relieving a number of different symptoms. Drinking chilled water actually cannot properly cool down your body whenever you feel hot—such as after eating spicy food. Instead, what it does is push the cold to your interior and leads your internal heat to the surface, to your abdomen, or to your chest. What results is symptoms manifesting as headaches, hot chest, night sweats, restless sleep, abdominal gas or cramps, irritability, low energy, thirst, sluggish digestion, and loose stools.

The mere act of drinking warm or hot water on a regular basis will relieve these symptoms effectively.

Prevents the body from wasting energy. Liquids that are below 37 degrees Celsius cannot be easily metabolized by the body—this includes room temperature water. As a result our bodies are forced to work harder, wasting unnecessary energy in order to make the cold drinks warm enough for it to use. I say unnecessary because this is energy that could be better used elsewhere, such as for healing illnesses and increasing our immunity against illnesses.

Helps with keeping organs properly hydrated and functioning

at their best. Did you know that you can actually dehydrate your organs if you constantly drink cool or cold water? Since it contracts and slows down the functions of your organs, you are also unconsciously training your body to become more averse to drinking water simply because you're taking it at the wrong temperature.

You won't feel the effects of dehydration immediately as you have grown accustomed to drinking cold, but when you do make the switch to warm water—you'll start to feel thirstier, as if your organs are asking you for more. This is because they are being "reactivated" from the cold-induced slumber. If you want to make the switch permanent, expect this thirstiness to last for 15 days to a month.

Helps balance the body's external and internal body temperature after doing physical activities. After exercising it is best to avoid drinking cold water as doing so will shock your organs and impede in your body's natural cool down process. During exercise, your internal body heat actually surfaces, which is what causes the hotness you feel and the sweating it comes with. This also means that your interior has become a lot cooler.

By drinking cold water, you're actually adding to that already-cold interior and as such, your body is not able to properly return to its normal temperature balance. Drink warm water instead in order to aid this and protect your organs in the process is well. Just make sure it's warm and not hot so you can avoid sweating further.

For children experiencing stomachaches and constipation, drinking lots of warm water is the best solution. Most people would immediately reach for a cup of tea, but this does not count because caffeine contains a diuretic and does not have the same hydrating effect that water does. What you can do, to give plain water a bit of taste, is to add some lemon juice or a bit of honey.

TIP: If you already live in warm, hot, or tropical climates then your body's qi flows closer to the surface when compared to those living in colder climates. It is often enough for you to drink warm water as opposed to drinking hot water, which might be uncomfortable given that it will further warm you up.

REMOVING SUGAR FROM YOUR LIFE – MADE EASY

We tackled plenty in this lesson and you have certainly learned a lot. Now, it's time to apply everything you have learned to your life and start making the necessary changes to create holistic health.

Begin by getting rid of sugary drinks from your diet.

Understandably, if you're a big soda drinker, this can be hard. So what I intend to do is slowly ease you into the process. For the first week, I want you to simply focus and observe the drinks you're consuming. If possible, note it down so you have a more physical reminder. Write down what you drink in the morning and throughout the day. Do you find yourself purchasing drinks such as Minute Maid? What about energy drinks? Maybe you're always buying offee, hot chocolate, lemonade, milk shakes, boba teas, smoothies, or those refreshing slurpees from 7-11.

Now, I want you to look at what you have written and realize just how badly these things can be to your body. The way they can cause sugar spikes in your bloodstream and all of the consequences that come with that. Terrible, right? Next, I want you to start eliminating them from your diet. If you have any soft drinks or sugary beverages in your kitchen right now, pour them down the drain. Make sure you do this as swiftly as possible—dilly dallying can actually make you hesitate and even keep some for yourself.

Remember, it is detrimental to your health so by throwing them out, you're doing your body and your health a BIG favor.

After clearing up your fridge, it's time to put what you've learned about habits into action. I want you to start creating triggers so you end up drinking more water. Place a glass by your bed and all over the house where you spend a lot of time in. Carry a bottle in your work bag and in your gym bay. Buy yourself a reusable water bottle that you can bring with you everywhere. You can even add a few slices of lemon to it, if you still want that flavor but not the bad stuff that comes with it.

You can also use your reward test whenever you crave sugary drinks. Instead of going out to get some, go for a walk or call up a friend. If you want to attack the behavior itself and curb the craving, a tablespoon of coconut oil will do just that.

WORKSHEET:

This time, using your habit tracker from the previous module, we'll be tracking your progress when it comes to eliminating sugary drinks from your life. The same goes for developing the habit of drinking water more. Your tracker should look something like this:

HABITS	1	2	3	4	5	6	7
GET RID OF SUGARY DRINKS							
DRINK 6 GLASSES OF WATER							

WEEK 5:

BREAKFAST IS THE MOST IMPORTANT MEAL OF THE DAY—

Congratulations on making this far! In the previous module, you have learned a lot of rather surprising things about sugar. I hope you have also taken the necessary first steps in eliminating it from your life, starting with what you drink on a daily basis. Simply doing that can create significant changes for your overall health so don't hesitate when it comes to breaking this particular habit and replacing it with new ones. Yes, it won't be easy but it is certainly worth the effort.

This time, we will be tackling the "meat" of holistic weight loss.

In the next modules, you will be learning more about the different weight loss methods that will help improve your holistic health. These will aid you in laying down the proper foundation so you'll be able to sustain your progress for years and years. Typically, all the information needed for this can be so overwhelming, but I've made summarized all the essentials into what I call the "5 Golden Rules of Weight Loss".

If you can successfully manage these, you are well on your way to succeeding with your weight loss goals and improve your health even further.

THE 5 GOLDEN RULES OF WEIGHT LOSS

To summarize: What you need to do is cut out the really bad food in your life and replace these with better ingredients. Basically, take out the bad and replace it with what's good. Sounds simple, right?

REMOVE REFINED SUGAR. We tackled this in the last module and is the most obvious choice when it comes to removing things from your everyday diet. It doesn't really serve any nutritional purpose and yet you will gain plenty of good benefits once it's been removed. Start with your drinks, then move on to the snacks and your daily meals.

REMOVE WHEAT FROM YOUR DIET. This means cutting down on bread and pastries—along with other similar food products. We will discuss this further later, but it's best we lay down the facts at the beginning. Again, these don't have much nutritional value and can be replaced by something better and healthier.

KEEP IT SIMPLE. This means opting for simpler foods and removing processed ones from your diet. I'm talking organic and whole foods that have been grass fed and pasture raised. So many processed food products contain an abundance of sugar and a slew of other bad stuff like hydrogenated oils which are all detrimental to your health. Instead of picking and choosing the bad ingredients, go for the big one and just removed anything processed from your diet.

MAKE SURE YOU'RE EATING ENOUGH HEALTHY OILS AND FATS. This is important—remember not all fats and oils are bad for you. Some are needed by the body to sustain good health and serves a purpose in terms of nutrition and keeping the different organs functioning properly.

MAKE VEGETABLES A DIET STAPLE. This one needs no explanation—we all know how beneficial vegetables can be when it comes to our overall health. It's simply a matter of putting thought into action and actually adding more of it into our daily diet.

My goal is to teach you a way of revamping your diet through the "meal first" approach. This means that you will be building your new diet by tackling each meal first. Along the way, you will also be learning more about different nutrition concepts. In this way, you're both learning and applying that knowledge in real life—this is my way of keeping you from getting bored whilst making sure that every lesson sticks.

We will begin with breakfast, then move on to lunch and dinner meals. After which we will work on the snacks or any other small meals you eat in between of the big ones. Chances are, even your habits of snacking in between your meals will lessen or be completely eliminated given the recipes and prep meals I'll be providing you with are both healthy and filling.

We will still be making use of what you've learned about breaking and building habits, so keep those steps in mind as well.

GETTING STARTED:

Now that you know the key rules for weight loss and holistic health, let's focus on building a roadmap. We will be approaching this using a 3-step process that focuses on each of your main meals, one at a time. Keep in mind that we're trying to build new habits here and to do that, we must take things one step at a time.

So, what do you typically have for breakfast? The average American will have cereals, doughnuts or bagels—basically, something that involves wheat. Some people, however, don't even have breakfast at all. Out of all the aforementioned options, cereal is the most common according to a poll done by Good Morning America. The rest have some variety of pastry, whether that be at home or when they get to work.

I remember that before, at work, we got free bagels for breakfast every Friday. It was just a simple treat from the company, something that I used to look forward to. I enjoyed my pastries a lot and would never hesitate to get one for breakfast, lunch, and even dinner. It was back then when I used to think that a bagel or two was enough to satiate me until lunch. It was made out of wheat, after all, and wheat was supposed to be healthy and filling. Right?

It was only some years after that I realized the real reason why I felt hunger a little earlier than lunchtime. It was because of the wheat.

WHEAT ISN'T AS HEALTHY AS IT'S MADE OUT TO BE

Wheat, as you may already know, is one of the most common grains eaten by people globally. It comes from a type of grass called Triticum, which is grown in a number of different varieties to suit different needs. The primary species of it is common wheat or bread wheat, but you might also be familiar with other closely related species such as spelt, einkorn, durum, emmer, and Khorasan wheat.

We regularly consume white and whole-wheat flour in our everyday diet as these are key ingredients when it comes to baked goods such as bread and different pastries. Other wheat-based foods that people eat on a daily basis includes, noodles, pasta, bulgur, couscous, and semolina. As popular as it is, wheat is also highly controversial within the health-conscious community because it contains GLUTEN, a protein that can actually trigger a harmful immune response if you're predisposed to it. This is what people refer to as "gluten allergy".

We have discussed what our primitive ancestors used to eat and how they avoided eating grass because it produced ill effects in their bodies. It was only after a few thousands of years when people learned how to cultivate and eat the grass seeds which is how wheat eventually became part of our diets. It doesn't necessarily mean that this food is wholly good for us, however. Some studies do suggest that it can be a rich source of fiber, vitamins, minerals, and antioxidants for people who can tolerate it. But that's the keyword, isn't it? It's only good if you're one of those who can metabolize it properly.

You are already familiar with why wheat is popular among people, now let's talk about why it could be bad for you.

To keep things simple, it's bad because the wheat people are eating these days isn't the same strain as the one our ancestors ate before. In fact, within the past 50 years, the overall chemical structure of wheat has changed—it has mutated. These changes go past the physical, too. Unlike the tall grains in the past, ones that reached over 4.5 feet tall and can now only be seen in period movies such as Gladiator, the wheat we have today is under 2 feet tall and significantly hybridized. Something that has been done in order for big food companies to produce more of it for cheap.

Think of it this way, creating hybridized versions of wheat can be likened to a painter matching all the colors he has in an attempt to create something new, but because he has mixed way too much the painter has ended up with a disgusting color in the end. This is how big food companies tampered with the original strain of wheat. They mixed and matched different ones, trying to improve on its resilience, resistance to bugs, or trying to improve yield but because there's so many wheat varieties what they ended up is wheat that's been completely genetically modified. Very, very different from what people had thousands of years ago.

To put this into perspective, here are 3 of the major mutations found in modern wheat.

GLUTEN

This is something you might already be familiar with, given that it is rather controversial among the health and fitness community. Gluten serves the purpose of making your bread stretchy and doughy, but it must also be known that it wasn't in natural to the original strain of wheat. Gluten is a mutation and doesn't really provide our body any significant nutrients. Needless to say, it causes more harm than good.

PHYTATES

This is another mutation that was developed to help wheat become more resistant to pests. Given the fact that pests are some of the biggest culprit for crop destruction and major losses for the food industry, it only makes sense that they create a breed of wheat that contains plenty of phytates. At first glance, this might seem like a great thing. After all, the higher the supply then the more affordable the product will be, but the thing with phytates is that they actually hinder proper mineral absorption. This includes a lot of the essentials, such as iron, zinc, calcium, and magnesium. Needless to say, this often leads to deficiencies including skin rashes and anemia.

AMYLOPECTIN A

The third mutation you must know about is Amylopectin A. To better understand this, let's go back to our previous discussions where we talked about how grass isn't digestible by humans and by extension, the same goes for their seeds as well. That is until the seeds are crushed into little pieces—only then can we absorb and metabolize them.

In modern grains, Amylopectin A is a component that's super digestible—so digestible, in fact, that it can easily cause to raise our blood sugar levels to spike more than any other food can. Much higher than table sugar. But that's not all, it can also block your body from absorbing the important minerals it needs in order to stay healthy.

OTHER KNOWN MUTATIONS

We've talked about how the industry is after more yield and higher resistance in order to make more profits. What this means is that there are literally thousands of other proteins added to the wheat strain to protect it from pathogens; these are proteins that are not always good for our body and overall health.

This includes serpins, CoA oxidases, a-amylases—among other things. There are even fungal enzymes such as xylaneses, cellulases, and glucoamylases added to help enhance the texture of the wheat products. Needless to say, if you're looking for simple food, then this isn't it. Imagine taking all of those proteins, many unknown to you and with effects you're uncertain of, each time you consume wheat products.

Does it still seem appetizing to you?

WHEAT ADDICTION

Addiction? To wheat? You may or may not see it, but it can cause an addiction that's no different from those people have when it comes to cigarettes. It begins with digestion, which creates compounds that are similar to morphine. These would then bind itself to the brain's opiate's receptors thus making it feel a mild happiness, a kind of reward that it will begin to crave with constant stimulation.

Now, if this effect is blocked, people will experience withdrawal symptoms—usually very unpleasant ones. For example, after your blood sugar levels begin to drop, you get super hungry and even cranky! Ever hear of the word "hangry"? It is real and it happens as a withdrawal symptom produced by our brain that's craving the effects of wheat.

This is also why even after having a high-wheat breakfast, you still get those pre-lunch cravings. All of that is because of gliadin.

WHEAT CAUSES VISCERAL BELLY FAT

Among the slew of negative effects caused by wheat, this is one of the most annoying and most detrimental to your weight loss goals. How does it happen? Well, try and recall the previous module where we discussed the concept of your blood sugar increasing and how that's really bad for your body. Now, keep in mind that wheat can cause this as well and in a way that's a lot more significant than other carbs—this is due to its amylopectin A content. The most digestible form of glucose.

That whole wheat bread you believe is healthy? It can increase your blood sugar level more than sucrose can. In fact, eating 2 slices of it is worse than drinking a can of sugary soda or eating a candy bar. This is based on the glycemic index, which measures how much certain food can increase blood sugar in the body. The glycemic index for bread for instance is 69 while a Snickers bar only accounted for 41.

Now, the higher your blood glucose is after eating, the higher your insulin level is and the more fat is added to your body. If you continue on with this cycle, that fat goes straight to your belly, causing it to get bigger and bigger. This is why even if you're relatively thin, you might find that your belly still protrudes. It isn't because you lack exercise or need to do more crunches—it's because you have too much sugar in your diet.

The bigger your belly becomes, the more resistant it is to insulin. This puts you at risk of developing diabetes. The fat around your belly is actually referred to as visceral fat, it's different from other types of body fat and also causes much more damage to your body. What it does is produces and sends inflammatory signals to your body. It can also trigger a host of other health related issues including colon cancer, rheumatoid arthritis, and even dementia. This is what I mean when I say holistic health is important. Your belly fat alone can influence, not just your body, but your mental health as well. Everything is connected and as such, there needs to be a balance within the whole.

WHEAT CAUSES TOOTH DECAY

We've touched on this earlier, but this time we're going to tackle the nitty-gritty details as to how wheat can cause this. After all, weren't we told that it's candy and sugar that causes tooth decay? Recalling what you have learned so far, however, you already know that sugar isn't just contained in all things sweet. It can also be found in your pastas, in your noodles, your whole wheat bread, and other similar food items.

It's the phytates in these that causes tooth decay. Because it blocks the body's efficient absorption of different nutrients and minerals from the food we eat, we end up experiencing deficiencies. A good example of which is Vitamin D deficiency which essential for our body to absorb calcium, especially in our teeth. Because it cannot absorb calcium from our food, the body winds up taking it from our bones and teeth—causing them to become brittle, which then leads to tooth decay.

In fact, a study done by Nature Genetics proves that cavities become more prevalent after grains were introduce into our diet. These scientists looked at the oral bacteria that causes cavities in human skeletons ranging from 100 to 6000 years old. They found that the rate of problematic oral bacteria increased significantly during the time humans began farming—introducing a change in our oral ecosystem and causing tooth decay.

TO RECAP:

Wheat can worsen tooth problems and inhibit your body from absorbing essential minerals for bone and teeth health.

It can also cause cravings, which is detrimental to your weight loss goals. It can also become addicting, messing with your brain, and the blood sugar levels in your body.

THE MISCONCEPTION WHEN IT COMES TO GLUTEN-FREE FOOD

In the previous lesson, you learned more about the negative effects that wheat has on the body. Now, we're going to tackle a key misconception that most people have when it comes to it.

I'm sure you've seen plenty of gluten-free labeled products at the grocery store and it is likely that you also know a few friends or acquaintances who follow a gluten-free diet for weight loss and health. There's a whole lifestyle dedicated to avoiding gluten, believing that in doing so they are living a healthier life. However, many still wonder why they keep gaining weight despite avoiding products that contain gluten.

Then you have gluten-free food.

Fact is, whilst these food products are indeed gluten-free, they do contain some form of replacement. Instead of wheat flour, you get rice starch, cornstarch, tapioca starch or potato starch. So even if they have taken out the gluten component and will no longer trigger an immune response from those who have the allergy, these food products remain bad for your overall health. This is because they are still capable of increasing your blood insulin by a whole lot. And as you already know, regular increases in your blood sugar levels can lead to really bad side effects.

What's worse is that these gluten-free replacements are capable of raising your blood sugar at a higher level than wheat can. So with wheat already passing soda and candy bars in terms of raising your blood sugar, can you imagine just how devastating these alternatives can be? Needless to say, you're replacing something bad with something that's also bad, but in a different way. Both can easily damage your body and health with continuous consumption, too.

The bottom line here is simple: You have to remove both wheat and gluten-free products in your diet because both have bad effects on your body.

WHAT ABOUT THE OTHER GRAINS?

Not all grains are created equal, this is a fact. Things like barley and rye both have a similar genetic history with wheat, as such they also have some of the bad effects that wheat has. That said, there are also non-whet grains such as oats millet, chia seeds, and so on. These are essentially carbs that don't bring about the bad immune or brain effects that wheat has. Consuming these in moderation is actually good for the body.

Another great grain option is flaxseed. This mainly comprised of fiber, oils, and protein. It is free of carbs that increase blood sugar levels. It can be a great alternative to your usual wheat based cereals.

THE KEY TO MEAL PREPPING

In our previous lesson, you learned more about the dangers of wheat and how it has since mutated from the ones your grandmother used to put in her cookies. With that new information in mind, we can begin changing up the meals you take each day—starting with breakfast. This is the most important meal of the day and is also when we consume most of the wheat in our diets. Think cereals, bagels, whole wheat bread toast, and so on. Once you drop all of that, what else can you have during the mornings that will provide you with energy but without the blood sugar spikes?

SAMPLE BREAKFAST OPTION: WHAT I HAVE EVERY MORNING

As I've discussed earlier, I like to keep my food and meals as simple as possible. For breakfast, I would usually have two boiled eggs, a spoonful or two of ground almonds, half and avocado, some flaxseed, and some walnut. Of course, I always have my morning cup of coffee with cream and some grass fed butter and coconut oil. That provides me with ample energy so I get a head start on my tasks every morning. If you don't drink coffee, however, you can skip that and take a teaspoon of coconut oil and butter instead.

Some days, when I'm not in a rush, I would have some overnight oats topped with blueberries. I also add flaxseed, walnuts, strawberries, and almonds to my yogurt. These are all easy to prepare and would only take a few minutes out of your morning routine—but they also make for the healthiest, wheat-free breakfasts that you can have. The best bit is that these aren't that expensive either compared to your usual bagel or cereal meals.

The key detail here is meal prepping. As the name suggests, this is basically the process of making our meals beforehand. In this lesson, I'll be providing you with an introduction to it—an easy to follow step by step guide that you can practice for a week or so. What you need to remember here is to keep things simple and convenient for yourself. Also, choosing the right ingredients counts when it comes to how effective your meal preps are

So, going back to my breakfast. I don't spend too much time on it—in fact, I have my eggs pre-cooked from the day before then simply proceed to making my instant coffee. Then I eat a spoonful of the seeds and the nuts. Takes about 5 minutes and I can continue with the rest of my morning routine. All of that can keep me sated for the entire morning until lunchtime rolls around.

That, friends, is reliant on the ingredients I have chosen for my breakfast. We'll cover this later as not all breakfast foods would provide you with the same energy or keep you sated for hours.

MEAL PREP AND ITS BENEFITS

Meal prepping can be compared to lunchables or bento boxes where everything is prepared ahead of time and all you really need to do is bring one along with you. Unlike those two, however, you have full control over your meal preps because you'll be making them yourself.

There's plenty of benefits to doing this, aside from the fact that it is very convenient.

First, you're able to save money. This is because you can now buy things in bulk which is always cheaper than buying food piece by piece. There's also a lower likelihood of you overbuying things because you already know what you need and how much of it you have to get. Eating out can be very expensive and if you do it every single day, those numbers can add up. Not to mention the fact that the food at these restaurants isn't always healthy—especially if you go for fast food each time.

Second, it supports your weight loss goals. Think back to the 3 components of behavior we studied previously: ability, trigger, and motivation. Meal prepping aids you when it comes to your ability to make healthier choices when it comes to everyday meals. It takes out the thinking process, primarily. This is because you now have a system in place and you can group your tasks together, lessening the chances of you feeling overwhelmed. It's pretty much setting aside a day to finish all your meal preps and you're good to go for the next 6 to 7 days. That's a LOT of time saved and a LOT of stress off of your shoulders.

Also, plenty of good meals to be had without needing to worry about it being a detriment to your health or weight loss goals.

THE ESSENTIALS – MEAL PREP PANTRY

Alright, for beginners, figuring out the proper staples for your meal prep pantry can be quite confusing. What do you need to buy? What's a non-essential that you can skip? Knowing these things, among others, can actually make meal prepping a smoother process. If you have everything you need within arm's reach, not only will you be more motivated to do the prep, but it's also easier to get inspired about what else you can make.

With that in mind, here's a list of pantry essentials that every meal prepper should have:

Spices. Now, this can get a little pricy and if this is your first time meal prepping then I suggest you stick to the basics. Stock up on:

Salt

Pepper

Garlic powder

Onion powder

Cinnamon

Chili powder

Cumin

Oregano

Ground coriander

Cayenne

Basil

Oils, sauces, and vinegars. The best bit about these is how versatile they can be. I have used them on salad dressings, flavoring dishes, making granola bars, energy bites, and even added them in certain drinks. Stock up on:

Coconut oil

White wine vinegar

Olive oil

Apple cider vinegar

Reduced sodium soy sauce

Balsamic vinegar

Worcestershire sauce

Sesame oil

Maple syrup (take in moderation)

Dijon mustard

Honey (take in moderation)

Organic lemon juice

Natural peanut butter

The pantry basics. This list is pretty basic and is mostly meant for preparing meals in a pinch. The key here is to get things that can either be eaten by itself or mixed together.

Rolled oats

Steel cut oats

Almonds

Walnuts

Flaxseeds

Quinoa

Chia

Almond butter

Regular grass fed butter

Eggs

Coconut oil

Cocoa or organic chocolate chips

Corn kernels

Chickpeas

Black beans

Mung beans

Full fat coconut milk

Almond milk

Soy milk

Chicken stock

*Note that these can be tweaked according to your preferences and the type of meals you're most likely to make. Just keep in mind all of our previous lessons and make sure that you avoid sugar and wheat products.

CHOOSING CONTAINERS

When you meal prep, one of the key things you cannot overlook is storage. Not only does it need to be organized, the meals you prepare also need to stay as fresh as possible—you wouldn't want to waste hours of work on something that ends up spoiling before you can even eat it. Whilst it might be tempting to reuse something like old cheese containers, it is still best to invest in something that will help reduce the chances of spoilage, is microwavable, is safe for food storage, and will be leak proof since you are keeping these for quite a bit of time in your fridge.

Here's what you need to consider when choosing good meal prep containers:

Air-tight and leak-proof lids. This goes for both storage and bringing food out with you. The last thing you want is to find that your breakfast or lunch has managed to spill of its container—that's time and money wasted in a flash.

In my opinion, snap-on lids aren't the best. However, if you can find one that comes with a suction seal or a lock mechanism that keeps the lid firmly closed even if you toss the container around then I'd say that's the one. Also, always test the product before purchasing it. Just because it looks air-tight, it doesn't mean that it will be. Give it a shake, lean it on its side, and wait for gravity to do its thing.

Plastic? Probably a no-go. Look, I get it, plastic is cheap and cheerful. It's also convenient since it's light and easy to carry around. However, they aren't always safe for food storage or for microwaving. See, some are simply not meant for that job. Have you ever experienced the displeasure of discovering melted plastic in your microwave after you tried heating food?

Then there's also the fact that it could leak all sorts of nasty chemicals into your fit whilst it's being heated. Sure, it can withstand the microwave, but let's not overlook the bad stuff that could be transferred to our food in the process. In my opinion, glass containers are the safest option. Sure, they're a little heavy —but that's a small price to pay to make sure you're eating good food. You have put in all of that effort, after all.

Freezer friendly. As with any meal prep, you're going to have to freeze your food in order to ensure its longevity. That means you'll be exposing it to sub-zero temperatures which can easily result in freezer burn if you're not using the right containers. Note that improperly kept frozen food items will also absorb other flavors and smells—truly terrible.

This is why you need to get freezer-friendly containers that will protect your food from freezer burn and make sure it retains the right texture, and flavor. Glass ones are the best, along with mason jars, but do make sure you give it enough allowance for your food to expand and crystallize. Ziploc bags are great alternatives as well, if you're looking for something a bit more space-efficient.

*Note: Always check the expiration periods for every ingredient that you use in your meal preps; this is especially so if you're not planning on eating them within the same week you made them.

YOUR FIRST MEAL PREP – A STEP BY STEP GUIDE

Now that you know the basics of meal prepping, I'll walk you through making your first meal that should last you about 5 days. That's 5 days of not having to worry about what to eat or what to make.

Ingredients:

Half an avocado

2 eggs (pasture raised and grass fed)

Instant organic coffee

A spoonful or two of flaxseed, almonds, and walnuts

Extra virgin coconut oil (1 tablespoon for the coffee)

Organic grass fed butter (1 tablespoon for your coffee)

Instant organic coffee

These are ingredients that you can easily get at any supermarket. As much as possible, however, do find organic varieties or buy them in bulk from places like Whole Foods. Now, I know that you're already thinking that these could get expensive—and trust me when I say that this is also one of the reasons why I hesitated on making the switch at first as well. Money can be a real issue when it comes to eating healthier as the ingredients can be a lot pricier compared to your usual fast food fare.

However, when compared to the cost of getting sick investing money into eating healthier is the cheaper option. Besides, your take outs do add up as well, especially if you eat it every single day. Whereas if you buy food in bulk and meal prep, you only have to spend a certain amount of money once and rest easy for the following week or two. Think of your food as medicine and that you're investing hard-earned money into making sure that your body is getting the best possible one in order to stay healthy.

Understandably, you might also be worried about time. The average person and your typical student would only have about 20 to 30 minutes of free time each day in order to get things done before they need to leave. So, how do they fit meal prepping into that tight schedule? Worry not, we shall tackle that as well. As always, the key is to make things simple to make it easier for you to incorporate this new habit into your lifestyle. Again, we shall be putting the habit system into play.

So, let's figure out how to deal with the cost of healthy ingredients.

One of the first things you need to do is look up bulk food stores and farmers markets around your area. It doesn't matter if they're the pop-up kind where they only open on weekends. The point here is to stock up on what you need at a price that's lower than what's available at your local grocery. Buy only what you need so you don't end up with food waste as well. For $15, which is the cost of about 3 to 4 take-out meals per day, you could get plenty of fresh produce and fruits to add to your diet. If you double that, you'll have more than enough supply for a week or even two of food.

It's all about making small sacrifices and really quitting your fast-food lifestyle.

Next, let's talk about making time. This is one of the harder challenges, but it certainly isn't impossible to accomplish. Do you have an hour or half an hour to spare? If you do, that's enough time for you to finish a few meals; maybe 3 to 4 depending on what recipe you're following and the ingredients you're using. If you have a bit more money to spare and if you don't have it already, investing in a food processor will help you cut down on even more time. You can finish grinding nuts or even veggies within a few minutes then you're good to go. These sell for about $25 or even less on Amazon. If you can borrow one from friends (if they're not using it) or your parents, do it!

YOUR 30-MINUTE MEAL PREP GUIDE

Prepare the night before:

Boil 10 eggs. Once done, store them in a container.

Grind your nuts and seeds, about a month's worth of it.

These two tasks shouldn't take up too much time and can actually be done between all of your other chores.

Come morning, all that's left to do is boil some water for your coffee. After, cut open your avocado then take out 2 of the eggs. You can even opt to cut small slabs of butter or coconut oil the night before, but since these are super minor details, you can do it on the day itself.

And that's it, you're done with your first meal prep.

If you want something different, you can also follow this oat-based meal prep.

Prepare the night before:

Soak your overnight oats.

Soak your seeds.

Come morning, you can drain the water from your oats and toss it in a blender along with the seeds. Add some yogurt, some almond milk, and maybe a squirt of honey. Pulse this until it becomes like a smoothie then top with some blueberries. That's it, your healthy breakfast oat-based smoothie. This should take you no more than 15 minutes to do.

As for clean up, it'll be a breeze since you're not using too many tools or containers. Consider that as well when you're prepping. The less tools, the simpler your prep is, the easier to clean.

ASSIGNMENT:

Your assignment for this module is to figure out your first week of breakfast and get the ingredients. I suggest you start simple and use my examples above. Not only are the ingredients cheaper, they're also easier to find and work with, without scrimping on nutritional value.

Once you're done with that, create another habit tracker. This time, replace your bad breakfast habits with this new one. Your tracker should look similar to this:

	1	2	3	4	5	6	7
GET RID OF SUGARY DRINKS							
DRINK 6 GLASSES OF WATER							
ELIMINATE WHEAT PRODUCTS							
HEALTHY BREAKFAST							

WEEK 6:

BREAKFAST AND NUTRITION—

So, how did your first week go? Were you able to keep up your new habit? Don't worry if you slipped up a few times, you'll get the hang of it if you just continue on.

In this lesson, we will be discussing more about breakfast nutrition and why I chose those specific ingredients for the recipe I shared with you. As you already know, breakfast is the most important meal of the day and it needs to provide you with as much energy as possible so you don't end up getting hungry before lunch time.

This week, we will be learning more about key ingredients, their nutritional value, as well as setting up the proper foundation for the other meals you need to work on as well. There's still lunch and dinner, after all.

THE MISCONCEPTION ABOUT FRUITS

For many people, fruits are a staple breakfast food. Many of us would either have an apple or two in the morning instead of a regular breakfast. Whilst there are others who would top their cereals, oats, pancakes, and yogurts with a variety of fresh and dry fruits. However, what many don't realize is that not all fruits can be consumed in unlimited qualities. Yes, they are healthy, but we must still practice moderation when it comes to them.

MUTATED FRUIT

Much like wheat, the fruits we have today have been highly hybridized, causing many different mutations and changes to its overall composition. Some contain more sugar than others, whilst there are ones that don't provide much by means of nutrients.

So how much fruit can we eat? This depends on the type you're eating. 1 serving of each kind should be plenty for every meal, even if you're only having it as dessert. You also need to look into a particular fruit's sugar content in order to make sure that having it regularly won't cause your blood sugar levels to spike unexpectedly.

As always moderation is always key, if you're unsure.

What you should really stay away from are fruit juices. This includes fruit juices that have been extracted from the fruit itself —they are simply not good for you and are actually overloaded with sugar. In fact, you are drinking more of the sugar instead of the actual fruit juice. In some cases, the flavor of the fruit is artificial so you're basically drinking liquid sugar.

In the case of dried fruits, whilst these have large amounts of antioxidants their high sugar and calorie content completely trumps all the benefits it could provide. If it can't be helped, having a few pieces with your yogurt should be enough—but always consume these in small amounts. Some people tend to snack on these thinking they are healthier replacements for the usual chips, but what they don't realize is that they are overloading their bodies sugar in the process.

THE GOOD AND THE BAD ABOUT FATS

One of the first things you might have noticed about my breakfast plan is that it contained grass fed butter and coconut oil. I'm sure you're thinking—fat is not good. You might have also thought about why I asked you to put it into your coffee instead of adding it to your meal. It sounds strange, yes, but I have a very good reason for asking you to do this. I want you to include healthy fats into your diet and those two are some of the best to include in your everyday meals.

We've already tackled the concept of bad fat versus good fat. How fat in general has been demonized, especially during the low fat movement of the 70s. You have also been fed many wrong information about it, especially by published studies that were covertly sponsored by big food companies. Again, many of these studies are just propaganda to promote the cheaper and less nutritious food that these companies are trying to get people to purchase.

Here's what I want you to remember: NOT ALL FAT IS BAD.

In fact, you need some of it in your daily diet to aid in proper brain function. That said, what's the difference between fats and oils? The simplest explanation is this: fats are the solid form and oils are the liquid version.

VITAMINS AND FATS

There are four different kinds that you need to be familiar with:

Saturated fats. This includes lard, cheese, healthy grass fed butter, and meats. 50% of your everyday consumption should come from these.

Mono saturated fats. This includes peanuts, olive oil, avocados, and almonds.

Polyunsaturated fats. These come from walnuts, fish, and flaxseed.

Cholesterol. This comes from butter, liver, eggs, and fish.

Then, you have your vitamins. I'm sure you're already familiar with this—you take vitamin c for colds or vitamin d to help with calcium absorption. Even from a very young age, you have been taught about the importance of vitamins in your diet. It is a nutrient that your body requires in order for it to continue functioning properly.

There are 2 Types:

Water soluble vitamins. This includes the likes of vitamin c and vitamin b. These are absorbed into our body along with water and if you consume too much of it, you'll just excrete it through your urine.

Fat soluble vitamins. This includes vitamins a, d, e, and k. These require fat so that they could be absorbed into our bodies. So, this means that if you're not consuming enough healthy fats in your diet, these vitamins don't get activated.

Think of it this way: These vitamins are vehicles of nutrition, but without a driver to help them get to the different places of your body where they are needed they remain stuck and are rendered useless. In this case, healthy fats and oils are your driver. They help the vitamins get to where they need to be and make sure that they are fully used by the body.

Without healthy fats in your diet, it doesn't matter how much calcium you get—your body won't absorb it because you don't have the right fats to activate it for you. Everything needs to work together in order to be effective and produce the results that you want.

Let's break that down further, shall we?

You need A and D, but to activate these two, you require K2.

A, D, E, K, magnesium, and zinc all work together.

Vitamin D is the calcium delivery truck which brings the nutrient to every part of your body that needs it. Without it, even if you take a ton of calcium rich foods, those are rendered useless. The same goes for taking calcium supplements. If your body is vitamin d deficient, it will not be able to utilize the calcium you consume.

Vitamin K2 helps make sure that the calcium stays out of your blood vessels.

How much vitamin D do you need to consume per day? For it to be effective, you should take 1000 IU per day. You can supplement this with 5,000 to 10,000 IU per day.

THE MOST COMMON MINERAL DEFICIENCIES

MAGNESIUM

Magnesium acts like an activator in our bodies. To be specific, it's the catalyst for 300 different chemical reactions. It powers these things in the same way a battery powers a car. In fact, vitamin D and vitamin A rely on magnesium so that they may carry out their different functions properly. And of course, vitamin D is also needed for a whole list of other processes--- including delivering calcium to the different parts of the body. Magnesium is essential to all of that so if you're low on it, these processes will not be performed properly and your body cannot function at its peak.

Magnesium is the easiest mineral and most commonly depleted minerals due to grains. This is why you require about 400 to 500 mg of it per day. Your natural sources for magnesium include: avocado, spinach, bananas, and black beans.

ZINC

Zinc helps with maintaining the structural integrity of protein. It aids the body in processing vitamin and supports the transport of other fat-soluble vitamins across the intestinal wall. The best natural sources for zinc includes food like mushrooms, chicken, spinach, chickpeas, lamb, and beef.

VITAMIN D

Among the 3, this is one of the most common deficiencies that people experience—especially for young children and teenagers. This is very strange considering the fact that we can easily get vitamin D from sunlight. However, times have certainly changed a lot from when humans were regularly spending time outdoors —whether that be for hunting or simply wandering about. They always got ample sunlight so there were never any deficiencies.

These days, however, most of us spend our days indoors. We work in air-conditioned buildings and we stay covered, away from the sun during the day. On weekends, we rarely see people spending time outdoors. Children prefer to stay inside, playing on their phones or computers. Young adults spend more time liking posts on social media instead of walking around in nature. Needless to say, we're not getting ample sunlight—hence the deficiencies.

What makes vitamin D important?

It's vital for a lot of important bodily processes, including brain function, the immune system, and metabolism. In a way, it influences the entire body so if there's a lack of it, the whole body feels the effects of it. We get inflammations more easily, we gain weight faster, we're more prone to spikes in our blood sugar, and we also heighten our risk for developing depression as well as cancers. This is because without vitamin D, our immune system is greatly compromised.

The best natural sources for vitamin D would be to sunbathe for about 30 minutes a day. This should be done before 8am as the sun is just hot enough and poses no danger to our skin during those hours. If you're not comfortable with sun exposure, you can also opt to get it through animal products such as liver and fatty fish. Egg yolks also contain plenty of vitamin D.

WHAT YOU NEED TO KNOW ABOUT GOOD AND BAD FATS

We have touched on this subject previously, but we shall be diving deeper into all the nitty-gritty details in this lesson.

One of the best types of fat that you can get is OMEGA 3. This is also why having fish in your diet is very important—but not just any type of fish. The best types to include in your diet are deep sea ones, such as:

Salmon (4,023 mg per serving)

Mackerel (4,107 mg per serving)

Herring (3,181 mg per serving)

Cod liver oil (2,664 mg per serving)

Sardines (2,205 mg per serving)

Anchovies (951 mg per serving)

Oysters (565 mg per serving)

You also have your nuts, which are also great sources of good fats. Raw ones such as pecans, almonds, and pistachios are great as everyday food. These can also serve as snacks if you're looking for something healthy and will boost your brain power. These contain a lot of fiber and can even lower your blood pressure. They key thing you need to remember is that they should be raw. Not baked, not fried—RAW.

Eggs and meats are okay, too. These can be healthy sources of fat for as long as you source them right. Grass fed livestock is the best as these have a much higher omega-3 fatty acid content. The fact that they are grass fed also means that they will not contain any antibiotics and growth hormones given to farmed livestock. Remember, these hormones and antibiotics aren't removed during meat processing and they end up in our bodies after. The same goes if you're drinking milk from bad livestock sources.

For cooking, use extra virgin coconut oil, avocado oil, or extra virgin olive oil. Did you know that these are so good for the body that you can have them in nearly unlimited qualities? The best bit is that these have a flavor on their own which only enhances that of what you're cooking. I mean, even Italians use olive oil for dipping. You can use these oils in a variety of ways as well. Add coconut oil to your drinks! Use avocado oil or olive oil for salad dressings! You can get really creative, without worrying about bad side effects.

If we're talking about the GOOD, we must also talk about the BAD.

It's simple really, you need to cut the following bad oils from your diet: corn, safflower, sunflower, grapeseed, cottonseed, soyben, fried oils, and hydrogenated oils.

AVOID VEGETABLE OIL. Big food companies often push the use of vegetable oils forward; products such as sunflower oil, canola oil, and corn oil are said to be healthier but—are they really? The thing is, they are very cheap to manufacture and very affordable for the average consumer, but the process of extracting these oils involves a VERY high heat process called hydrogenation. This exposure to high heat makes the oils very unstable and reactive in our bodies, and can often cause inflammation.

Lastly, I advice that if you're ever cooking using meat, it is healthier to use the whole animal. Look, I get it, the idea is unorthodox for some people but if you look at some of the healthiest countries in the world (particularly in Asia), they use the entire animal for eating. They have organ bone broth that's not only chockfull of nutrients, but also helps with boosting your energy and brain power. It's a dish that the whole family can enjoy.

IMPORTANT FACTS ABOUT DAIRY

Dairy is not just a staple in most pantries, they also tend to be a favorite for many people. Dairy is versatile and can be consumed in many different ways, but the first thing you need to remember is this: it is grayer than other foods and must be consumed in moderation. Secondly, not all dairy products are created equal. For example, it is okay to consume more of dairy products such as cheese when compared to others such as butter, yogurt, or milk.

Going back to the concept of KISS, you should choose dairy products that were leased processed. In this case, cheese is the least processed of the lot. Another thing to remember is that you should choose full fat, unflavored and unsweetened yogurt over one that has already been flavored in some way. The best thing to do is look at the ingredients list. I know it's easy to get tempted into purchasing the strawberry or blueberry flavored yogurts, but remember: SUGAR IS BAD. Worse than fat, in fact.

As for milk, always go for whole milk.

Traditional Chinese medicine states that dairy can increase dampness and phlegm—keep that in mind and make sure that you always consume dairy products in moderation.

SOY

This is another gray area when it comes to food, so I suggest that you soy in moderation. Much like milk, it also comes in a variety of different forms. It is recommended that you consume this in its fermented varieties such as natto, miso, and tofu because the fermentation process actually degrades the phytates and lectins it contains.

LEGUMES

Legumes are comprised of different bean varieties which are good to have in your diet—but much like soy and milk, do so in moderation. Favorites such as kidney beans, Spanish beans, black beans, and lima beans are all very easy to incorporate into any meal so they're good to have in your pantry. They also contain a lot of fiber and protein, but note that their carb content can become excessive if consumed in larger quantities.

WEEK 7:

MEAL PREPPING LUNCH—

By now, you probably have spent a good few weeks getting into your new breakfast habit. Congratulations on making it this far! This time, we'll be discussing lunch and how you can tweak it in order to fit your new, healthier lifestyle. Before we proceed, however, I just want to remind you that if you feel as if you need more time to develop each of the habits we've been discussing, feel free to do so! Take your time with it and don't feel as if you have to move on to the next step as soon as possible.

Remember, building habits is not a race. It will take time if you really want something that will stick for life.

Alright, back to lunch. What have you been having these days? For a lot of people, the answer is still the same: fast food. Look, I'm not here to judge you but I also want you to know that it really isn't good for you. Perhaps you've also been heating up a lot of packaged frozen food as well? Some hot pockets? I've been in your shoes before and I understand the difficulty of trying to find time for prepping and cooking for lunch. It isn't exactly as simple as breakfast.

However, it can be made more convenient so that you can incorporate it into your daily life.

First, I need you to make simple changes. Let's begin with cutting out processed food from your diet.

WHAT ARE PROCESSED FOODS?

Processed foods is basically any type of food—made more complicated. Anything that contains a bunch of ingredients, with names that you don't recognize. Think of it this way: an apple is just an apple. A chicken is just a chicken. A pack of Oreos is made up of many different ingredients aside from just a simple cookie and cream. The same goes for your usual pack of potato chips. It isn't just potatoes; there's a whole bunch of other stuff in there such as vegetable oils that are real bad for you. All hidden and packaged neatly to make everything more discreet.

Your frozen dinners? Those are processed foods as well.

PROCESSED FOODS: THE BAD AND THE UGLY

Packaged food is convenient, cheap, and it can also taste quite good. This is what I learned after I began living on my own—no mother to prepare and cook my meals for me. Independence was exhilarating until I realized that I had to do everything on my own now. I had to make my own food, clean up after myself, and all that not-so-fun stuff. It wasn't long before made food delivery and take out my best friend. At the supermarket, my go-to was the frozen food aisle. Anything that I could simply pop into the microwave, I got.

My diet consisted of—you guessed it—frozen dinners, frozen pizzas, burgers, pastas, and the occasional salad or fruit. I say occasional because these can be expensive and I was on a very tight budget given that I had only started working. Back then, I didn't really prioritize healthy food—I just wanted fast and delicious things that would satisfy my hunger and make me feel good after a long day at work.

That was before I began talking to a friend who is quite knowledgeable about nutrition. She immediately noticed the change in my appearance, even though we haven't seen each other in a while. She pointed out my pallid complexion, my weight gain, and my fat belly. Yes, I was offended, but that was replaced with worry when she pointed out all the complications I could develop if I continued on with my diet.

Needless to say, I got scared.

But, see, I was not my mother and I wasn't at all skilled when it comes to cooking. I could fry or boil an egg—that's about it. I didn't want to give up, however. Look, I didn't want to die young—like I told you, I had many plans and if I were to achieve those then I had to stay healthy. So what I did was learn more about my options. That's when I stumbled upon KISS.

KEEP IT SIMPLE, STUPID (KISS)

The name isn't the most charming, but it belies how effective this technique is. This is a design principle created by the US Navy back in the 60's. It teaches us that things will work better and at its peak if we keep it simple instead of going for something complex. Basically, simplicity should be the goal when it comes to design.

This is the concept I followed when I first began making changes to what and how I ate. I did my best to keep everything simple, from the ingredients that I added to even the tools that I used. What I needed for my meals, I had to have ready access to. This made everything simpler and less stressful for me to do. Can you imagine needing to puree something only to find out that you don't have the right tool for it? It is likely that you'll delay doing it or give up altogether.

Work with what you have and keep it simple.

I applied this same concept to eliminating processed food from my diet as well. It was challenging at first because I was making it difficult for myself. When I figured out a system that worked for me, everything became much easier.

BUY – COOK – STORE

This is the simple formula that I used. I came to the realization that I always went for packaged, processed food because of its convenience. Once I set myself up for the task of making something simple from fresh ingredients and storing leftovers for the following day, I began questioning why I didn't do this before. It was easier than first thought. It only ate up a good half hour of my time as long as I kept my recipes simple.

And that's the key: SIMPLE.

MEAL PREP LUNCH IDEAS

I know the whole idea can be pretty overwhelming—I've been there, remember? So in this lesson, I have put together lunch ideas that even beginners can easily accomplish. This is simple yet healthy. After all, lunch need not be complicated in order to be delicious. Even the easiest dishes can be just as scrumptious.

For this particular recipe, you'll need three ingredients:

Chicken

Organic frozen veggies

Healthy herbs

For the chicken, you would want to get several pounds of organic chicken thighs with the skin on them. For the veggies, frozen is fine but do make sure it is organic and contains carrots and peas. The healthiest herbs you can find and should stock up on are salt, pepper, oregano, and thyme. The last two go best with chicken and will really enhance its flavor. You wouldn't want to be scrimping on taste!

Two chicken thighs, with the bone in, is typically good for one meal. Some people eat a bit less and can only really finish one—but that depends on how big the chicken is. Season this as you see fit then bake at 365 degrees for 55 minutes. That's all you really need to do for the chicken before letting it cool a bit then placing it in a pyrex container for the fridge.

Come morning, simply add your veggies to the container then

reheat it. Your total time? An hour and maybe 15 minutes. You can bring this lunch with you to work as well. Want to add something more? You can toss in some sweet potatoes, rosemary, garlic, and olive oil alongside your chicken when you're reheating it. This could easily work as a quick dinner recipe as well, just tweak as you see fit.

If you're not keen on chicken, you can have nice baked salmon instead. The process is similar to that of chicken, minus the veggies. Instead, you would want something like celery and some string beans. Both of which can be easily bought from your local supermarket. To give your salmon a light sauce, a bit of grass fed butter and some garlic should suffice. A drizzle of lemon on top with a hint of your favorite herbs will help boost the flavor even more.

You can also opt to throw in some potatoes when reheating it, to add a bit more weight to your lunch.

WEEK 8:

EASY MEAL PREP DINNERS—

And so we have come to the final module. By now, you've already learned plenty about building the right foundation for holistic health. We have covered the different aspects, from mental to physical. You have also learned more about nutrition and all the different misconceptions about some of the things you thought you knew.

In this lesson, I'm going to further bulk up your knowledge on what food is good, what you should eat less of, and what you should completely avoid. In doing so, I also hope that you'll be able to make better choices when at the grocery—as well as when it comes to budgeting your time and ingredients for your meal preps.

As always, we are still following the KISS concept and keeping things as simple as possible.

FERMENTED FOODS

They may not always look the most appetizing and they may even have strange smells at times, but did you know that fermented foods are some of the healthiest? The process of fermentation actually removes plant defenses whilst also adding good bacteria that's beneficial for our gut. Fermented foods supply our bodies with beneficial bacteria that helps with keeping our gastrointestinal tracts healthy. This means it also aids in proper digestion, boosting our metabolism, and in the absorption of nutrients from our food.

It is also worth noting that the fermentation process produces many valuable nutrients such as biotin, thiamine, riboflavin, and the essential K2 vitamin.

Some of the best fermented foods that you should add to your diet, include: tofu, sauerkraut, kimchi, kombucha, miso, tempeh, and apple cider. The best thing about these ingredients is how versatile they are—you can easily add them to any meal as a side-dish and boost its nutritional value. Getting them isn't difficult either; all of these are available at your local supermarket and organic food stores. They're easy to find and quite easy on the pocket as well.

That said, let's talk recipe. For this particular dinner, you only need a few ingredients.

A block of tofu

Beef strips

Frozen veggies

Garlic

Soy sauce

Salt and pepper

This should only take you a few minutes. Start by stir-frying your beef and garlic together. Add your tofu after cooking the beef to your desired doneness. Season this and add a tablespoon or two of soy sauce—make sure you give it a taste before adding anymore. Lastly, toss in your frozen veggies.

After that, you just let it cool down before keeping it in a pyrex container and storing in your fridge. This should last you a couple of days, depending on the amount you cook. Reheating is a fairly quick job as well since you only really need to either microwave it or heat it up in a pan with some oil. Do whichever is more convenient—though the latter option does give it a bit more flavor.

BROTHS

Broths are simple and chockfull of nutrition. The only real downside is that it takes a bit of time to do. Think a couple or more hours in order to really get that flavor you want. That said, it can still be meal prepped—especially if you have a slow cooker. You can leave it to slowly cook over a few hours whilst you do household chores, work on school stuff, or focus on other tasks that need to be done.

But first, back to the basics. What exactly is a broth? This is a soup that's cooked with meat on the bones. I say it's one of the healthiest, despite the meat content, because it is high in collagen. Now, if you're not familiar with it, collagen is essential for the building structures of our joints, skin, and other connective tissues. It keeps us moving with flexibility and prevents our bones from rubbing against each other whenever we move.

Without collagen—well, just imagine that there'd be plenty of friction in our joints and a whole lot of pain.

Broths can help with that, aside from being great sources of fat soluble vitamins. The best bit is that you don't really need much in order to make it. You just need beef bones with some meat on it. Any butcher shop will know exactly what to give you if you tell them you're making a broth. The rest is just water, seasoning, and if you want extra flavor—you can opt to toss in a few veggies as well. However, only do so near the end of boiling your broth as you don't want these to end up soggy or mushy.

GRASS FED MEATS

Just as wheat is generally not good for us, the same can be said for animals that consume grains. The idea for feeding cattle with this came from WWII farmers who realized that they could quickly fatten up an animal by feeding it surplus grain. The reality of that is there's no nutritional value in grain other than it made the cow fat—the process itself is not natural. Since we're eating grain-fed cattle, we don't get the right nutrients we would have had it been grass fed.

This is why you have seen me use the label "grass fed" for anything that's dairy related. This is because grass fed meat has been proven to be a good source of essential vitamins and minerals. But whilst it's good for the body, it should also be eaten in moderation. The recommended daily serving is 5 ½ ounces of lean meat for a 2,000 calorie per day diet. If you plan on having beans or other protein-rich plant based food, you can eat less than the recommended 5 ½ ounces to balance everything out.

When it comes to beef, I like to keep it as simple as possible. This time, we're going for classic steak strips so you'll be needing 3 to 4 pieces. The thickness should be no more than half an inch to make it much easier to cook. All you really need to do for this is melt about a teaspoon of grass fed butter, add some chopped garlic to that, then toss in your beef and some chopped bell peppers. Cook until it's nice and soft before plating. On top, add healthy herbs and season to your taste.

This can also be refrigerated and eaten as lunch or dinner the following day. To reheat, simply use your microwave or your oven, depending on how much free time you have for that day. You can also opt to add a couple of tomatoes, a pickle, and some adzuki beans when you heat the beef up.

If I have a bit more time to spare, I usually make a quick salad to go with my beef strips instead. That's lettuce, chopped cucumbers, half an onion (sliced), some tomatoes, cheese, and topped with either balsamic vinegar or simple olive oil with salt and pepper. Think of it as a palate cleanser after the beef. It makes for a light yet filling lunch as well.

Simple, delicious, and very convenient to make.

CONCLUSION:

Holistic health and weight loss will always have to go hand in hand. This is especially so if you want all the positive changes to your body to last. Sure, starvation diets produce quick results but at what cost? How many times can you do it before your body sustains damages that it cannot easily recover from?

I get it, it's easy to turn your back on challenges—especially if it involves overhauling your lifestyle and getting rid of the habits you're so used to. I've been there before and I understand how we can sometimes become blind to the mistakes in our ways. But just because we have grown accustomed to something, it doesn't mean that it is the only method of doing things. It doesn't mean that we can make it even better, because we can. This is what this course is for.

I want you to realize your own power, first and foremost, to make all the necessary changes. This course? It's simply a step-by-step guide to bring you to point A to point Z. Think of it as your map, but also remember that everything else is up to you. You're going to have to push yourself to applying all that you have learned. There will be tough days. Days when you feel like you'll never get over the bad habits you have or days when you're lazy or too busy.

On those days, I hope you remember how far you have gotten simply by choosing to say NO to yourself—the one that wants to quit. A little push goes a long way when it comes building habits that will sustain your overall holistic health. Every little push you make adds up and contributes to your success.